Cancer

YOUR QUESTIONS ANSWERED

£L

Cancer

YOUR QUESTIONS ANSWERED

Dr Charles Dobrée

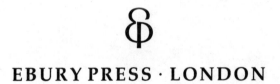

EBURY PRESS · LONDON

Published by Ebury Press
Division of The National Magazine Company Ltd
Colquhoun House
27-37 Broadwick Street
London W1V 1FR

First impression 1988
Copyright © 1988 Charles Dobrée

ISBN 0 85223 608 5

Senior Editor: Fiona MacIntyre
Editor : Miren Lopategui
Designer: Gwyn Lewis

Typeset by Text Filmsetters Ltd, London
Printed and bound in Great Britain at
The Bath Press, Avon

Contents

Notes: It must be emphasized that this book is intended merely as a general guide to the subject of cancer, and is in no way intended to be a substitute for professional medical advice. When in doubt, therefore, *always* consult your doctor.

Throughout this book, for 'he' read 'he or she'.

General Introduction

This book is one of a series designed to help you with a variety of medical problems. The overall approach that I am using in the series draws very much from my own personal experiences as a doctor. Over the years I have found one of the greatest problems in medicine to be a lack of communication between doctors and their patients. And although communication is a two-way affair, one of the most common complaints is that doctors do not communicate effectively with their patients. The importance of this cannot be over-emphasized. In order to achieve the best care in the shortest possible time it is essential that the doctor explain to his patient, in simple terms, the nature of the problem, how it is to be treated and what the consequences of the diagnosis and treatment are likely to be. And it follows that the more understanding a patient has about his disease the more successful the treatment is likely to be.

It is clearly important, therefore, that doctors fully inform their patients of the medical condition facing them. But in this respect a doctor is sometimes confronted by a basic problem. How does he know whether or not he has got his message across? How does he know if you, the patient, have fully understood the nature of your problem? Can he be sure that you appreciate the purpose of your treatment?

It is at this point that communication between doctor and patient often breaks down, simply because the doctor assumes that his patient has understood what has been said about his disease and appreciates the nature and purpose of the treatment.

Sometimes the only way your doctor will realize that he has not made himself clear is if you ask questions. Not only will this tell him that he has not made himself clear, it will also allow him, in answering your questions, to explain the particular points you have raised more fully, to satisfy himself that you have understood what he has said. It will also reassure him that he has really got his message across, for he will be only too well aware of the importance of understanding and co-operation from his patient. In addition, it may make him realize that his way of explaining a particular problem is, perhaps, not all that clear or helpful, and it will help him to improve his explanation of that problem to patients with a similar diagnosis in the future. In fact, doctors can learn a surprising amount by answering their patients' questions.

And this is really what this book is all about – directly answering your questions. In the following pages, you will find your questions in italics and my answers beneath them. So, without further delay, let's get into the book.

What's this book about?

This book sets out to answer your questions about cancer. In dealing with these questions I hope to dispel many of the myths surrounding this emotive subject. At the same time, however, I want to face some of the inevitable consequences of cancer in order to give as much helpful and practical advice as possible.

Containment of the problem is a practical possibility for most cancer sufferers. For everyone with the disease it is an imperative right from the moment of diagnosis. A positive and practical approach to the problem must, therefore, be adopted. Medical science may not know what causes some cancers and may not be able to completely cure them. But – and this is very important – it *can*, to a great extent, contain the problem and, with the full and positive co-operation of the cancer sufferer, can, in many cases, maintain a normal life span.

But can't my doctor answer these questions?

Of course he can, and I would not for one moment try to take his place. As a doctor myself I would feel very concerned if I discovered that one of my patients had had to turn to a book rather than approaching me directly with his questions. Throughout this book, therefore, you will find that I constantly advise you to consult your doctor if you have any doubts over any aspect of your particular problem.

Indeed, some of the answers that I give to your questions may themselves be unclear and you may need to clarify them with your own doctor. The real purpose of this book is to complement the advice that you get from your GP and consultant. The reason I think that you may need this help is because of the time factor. Often, doctors simply don't have enough time to explain all aspects of a particular problem to their patients. The main purpose of this book is to bridge that time gap.

In writing the book, I have collected together a large number of questions that I have attempted to answer over the years, and, sitting at my desk, have imagined that you are sitting with me and that we are having a normal consultation.

You are asking me questions and I am answering them. But the nice

2

thing about our particular situation is that we know that we are not going to have any interruptions, that if we feel like a natural break we can stop and take up where we left off. I am not suddenly going to have to disappear on an emergency call and you are not going to be made to feel uneasy because of restless and impatient noises out in the waiting-room.

There is also another important aspect: the problem of the spoken word. When discussing a particular problem with your doctor, it is often easy to miss something, and difficult, when you know that he is pressed for time, to ask him to repeat what he has just said.

One of the great things about having a book is that you can constantly refer back to it, thinking about what you have read and comparing it to what you have read in other books. In fact, reading a book is probably the best form of self-education there is. It is a form of learning and assimilation that can never quite be matched by the spoken word.

This book, then, is primarily an adjunct to what your doctor will already have told you, and provides a reference to what you have already learned about your problem. You may also find that it stimulates you to ask your doctor other questions. Questions that perhaps I have not raised in the book. But this is all to the good. The more information that you can acquire about your problem the better will be your understanding of it, and the better able you will be to set about coping with the problem.

Will I be able to understand the medical terminology?

Don't worry about this problem. Wherever possible I have tried to use uncomplicated words. When this has been unavoidable, I have either fully explained what the word means or have indicated that a definition may be found in the Glossary of Terms on pp.152-155. Apart from this general glossary, you will also find a Drug Glossary on pp.156-159 that explains how the specific drugs mentioned work and the various side-effects to be expected from them.

Terminology is a problem that is frequently encountered in the doctor–patient relationship. In particular, difficulties can often arise when trying to simplify what in some cases are complicated medical concepts. This is a trap that the most well-intentioned of doctors can easily fall into. Some doctors, in order to allay their patients' fears – feeling in some circumstances that the use of the word 'cancer' will be inappropriately alarming – use vague, nondescript terms such as 'ulcer', 'swelling', 'collection of fluid' and assume that their patients will, in the fullness of time, somehow come to understand the real nature of their problem. It is true that in special circumstances it is sometimes correct to withhold the specific diagnosis of cancer if it is felt that it will be too devastating a message, but a good doctor, if he knows his patient, should know exactly how and in what manner he should break this particularly unwelcome news.

In the main, however, I think that most doctors are of the opinion that it is best to tell their patients directly that they have cancer but at the same time to explain fully what this diagnosis means without using vague, undefined terms that may, in the long run, confuse rather than help. This can often simply lead to a total breakdown in communication between doctor and patient.

I hope that this book will, if needs be, fill this gap.

Is this a book only for people with cancer?

Although the emphasis of the book is placed upon cancer and the problems that arise from it, and is written primarily for those with the disease, it is also written with two other groups of people in mind.

One such group is the relatives of those with cancer. In the initial stages following the diagnosis of cancer it is often particularly difficult for relatives of the cancer sufferer to speak about the problem – especially if the cancer sufferer himself, for reasons that we shall go into, does not want to discuss his problem. I hope that this book will be helpful for such people for it will explain, in general terms, what cancer is all about. If you were not in the consulting room when your relative was told the diagnosis it will save you having to press him for details, at a time which may be particularly distressing for him, though, in the final analysis, as we shall discuss later, talking about the problem is a very important aspect of cancer containment. It will also help you to formulate the sort of questions that you would like to ask the doctor when, for instance, you accompany your relative for a subsequent consultation. Don't forget, doctors are always glad to answer your questions.

The other group of people this book is written for is the general public. Not just as a source of information – though I very much hope that this is what it will be – but also as a means of making everyone aware of what I believe to be a very important aspect in the battle against cancer; namely prevention and early detection.

In the following pages, advice on prevention and early detection of various cancers will be given. You will see, as you get into the book, that in most cases the earlier the cancer is diagnosed and treated the better the long-term outlook of containment of the disease actually is.

I hope that this advice will be of some value.

How should I read the book?

This book can either be read from beginning to end or, alternatively, can be dipped into. It is not one of those books that is dependent upon understanding what has gone before. Throughout, I have tried to keep the sections as independent from each other as possible, explaining and discussing the answers to each and every question as though that question were an entity in itself.

I think that probably the most benefit you will get from this book is to go through it fairly quickly, make mental notes of the parts that particularly interest you, and then read the sections that appear relevant to your problem more carefully.

The basic plan of the book is as follows.

Initially we will discuss the nature of cancer itself, what precisely it is and the various theories and factors that are thought to be responsible for its causation.

This section will deal with the scientific background to cancer and may seem slightly technical to some people. If you find this is the case, skip over it. A complete understanding of the scientific background to cancer is not necessary to appreciate the broader aspects of this book.

We will then discuss the clinical aspects of the common cancers and the ways in which they are investigated.

The fourth section will talk about the features and treatments of specific cancers. This is followed by a discussion of what is a very ignored aspect of cancer and its problems; namely, the social stresses thrown upon the patient and his immediate family. Included in this section will be a description of what it is like to be in a hospice. Finally, there is a Glossary of Terms, a Drug Glossary and a list of Useful Addresses (p.152).

What should I do if, when reading the book, I recognize a symptom or a feature that I think I may have?

If you do not have cancer but exhibit either a symptom or feature that is mentioned in the book, the most important thing is not to worry. The reason for this is as follows. The symptoms and features of many cancers are so nebulous that they can often resemble and mimic diseases and problems of no consequence. For instance, when I come to discuss cancer of the large bowel, you will see that a symptom of the disease is passing blood in the stools. Although this is a symptom of cancer of the bowel the most common reason for passing blood is haemorrhoids, also known as piles, which are simply little knots of dilated blood vessels that are found around the anal margin.

If you find that you are passing blood in your motions, therefore, the likelihood is that the problem is being caused by a bleeding pile rather than cancer.

Sometimes, when a loved one is ill or has died from a particular cancer, a caring relative might sooner or later develop symptoms which bear a strong resemblance to their loved one's illness. This is an example of a psychological response with no actual physical basis.

Both these examples are instances of how easy it is to jump to wrong conclusions, to assume that you have the symptoms or features of cancer. That is not to say that you should not take action, however. No symptom or clinical feature should be ignored. In other words, if, say, you find that you are passing blood in your stools, you should report this fact to your doctor, even though a simple examination will normally reveal a bleeding pile.

Do not ignore any symptom. Your doctor would far rather reassure you about a trivial problem than wait and have you come and see him with a serious problem that is at an advanced stage.

In short, as you read these pages, do not jump to any alarming conclusions. On the other hand, if the warnings do alert you to the possibility that you have a particular problem then, in the long run, time will have been saved in the treatment of your condition.

Is there a plan to the book?

The first part of this book sets out to tell you in general terms about cancer, its causes and how it is detected. Questions on specific cancers and their treatment are then answered and, finally, psychosocial problems of the condition are tackled.

This book is primarily designed as a practical guide to help all those with cancer, but is also written with the patient's friends and relatives in mind. It is often the friends and families of cancer sufferers who need as much support as the patient but who often feel isolated from the patient because they do not know enough about their friend or relative's problem.

A small book like this cannot hope to deal in detail with every single type of cancer and neither should it. As mentioned above, it will simply attempt to answer your questions about cancer in general terms. Various points will be discussed as they arise and illustrated with particular examples.

I shall concentrate on the more common forms of cancer, and shall explain in detail how such cancers can be both detected and treated, thus hoping to answer the general questions on diagnosis and treatment that are common to most cancer problems. For example, in discussing breast cancer I shall emphasize the principle of early detection by routine breast examination and will then show you how your doctor makes the diagnosis of breast cancer, the various tests that you may be submitted to, the various surgical procedures that you may be advised to undergo, the subsequent radiotherapy and chemotherapy and, finally, the nursing and counselling that are available. Although breast cancer is a specific problem, aspects of treatment underlying this condition are common to the therapies of many other cancers. Therefore, although your own type of cancer may not be dealt with in detail, I am sure you will nevertheless derive information that will be relevant to your particular problem.

What should I do if I find that advice in the book is at variance with my present treatment?

I hope that this problem does not arise. If it does, it is probably a result of my inability to explain myself clearly.

Throughout the book I have tried to describe and encapsulate present medical thinking but it is possible that by the time it goes to press, there will have been advances in therapy which, in some instances, may make what I describe seem obsolete. Whatever you do, whatever conclusions you draw from this book, it is important that you keep to the treatment that your doctor has prescribed for you. If a query does arise in your mind, jot it down on a piece of paper, then, the next time you visit your doctor discuss the problem with him. If needs be take the book with you to ask his opinion. Remember, doctors never mind being asked questions. Questions will help your doctor communicate with you.

What is cancer?

How does cancer arise?

Our bodies are made up of cells. Throughout our lives most of these cells are being continually replaced by a process of cellular division, in which each cell divides itself into two similar, 'daughter' cells. Each of these daughter cells, which has the same characteristics as the original cell, will, in turn, divide. This process of reduplication is called mitosis, and is taking place within our bodies all the time. Approximately every four months, for example, all our red blood cells are completely replaced by a new generation of red blood cells. Similarly, over a period of about eight months, all our old skin is shed, and replaced by a completely new layer.

We are unaware of this continual process of reduplication but it nevertheless occurs and does so for good reason. For tissues to remain functional, they must be composed of cells that are operating to their full potential. To take an example. Red blood cells have a very important role in that they carry oxygen to the various tissues in the body. As these cells age, however, their efficiency is impaired and they become less able to perform this function adequately. Now if there were no mechanism to replace these ageing red blood cells, all our tissues would soon become starved of oxygen. So this process of cellular renewal, revitalization and reduplication is the very foundation upon which our bodies remain in a healthy state.

In normal conditions, our bodies have evolved a delicate mechanism for controlling the rate at which new cells form and reduplicate. When, for reasons that we shall discuss later, this control mechanism breaks down, certain cells in the body begin to reduplicate in an uncontrolled way. It is when this happens that the problem is said to be cancerous.

To reiterate, then, cancer occurs when a small group of cells within normal tissue begins to reduplicate in an uncontrolled manner.

What causes cancerous cells to grow and divide unchecked?

This is a question that is of fundamental importance, but, unfortunately the complete answer still eludes us. The solution to the problem lies in a full understanding of the normal mechanism by which cells divide, and of the control mechanism which oversees cellular reduplication. The key to the whole question is probably to be found within the nucleus of the cancerous cell.

A normal cell has a nucleus which, in turn, contains genes. Genes are made up of a chemical called DNA, a complex protein whose full name is deoxyribonucleic acid. When a cell divides, it does so on instructions from its genes. In order for this to occur, the DNA receives chemical instructions to take up a particular configuration before initiating the process of division. It is probably in or around this chemical-controlling mechanism upon which the action of the DNA is dependent that the basic cause of cancer is to be found. It is thought to be at this level of chemical involvement that the DNA may sometimes receive disorganized and incorrect instructions. In other words, instead of being instructed to initiate the process of cellular reduplication in an orderly and regular way, it receives a garbled or incomplete set of chemical instructions, which makes it initiate cellular reduplication, but in a haphazard and uncontrolled manner, resulting in a mass of irregularly dividing cancerous cells.

What causes the chemical control mechanism of cellular duplication to malfunction?

This question takes us right to the very heart of the cause of cancer. Possible causes for the malfunction have been suggested by looking at specific sorts of cancer.

Let us, for the moment, go back to our original single cell and concentrate on the DNA in the nucleus. There are two basic influences upon this DNA. One is the influence that the DNA has upon itself, i.e. the genetic information that it contains. As a composite whole these are the genes – our hereditary blueprints, passed from generation to generation. In certain individuals, families and racial groupings, however, this genetic information can cause the reduplicating mechanism of the cell to malfunction. We often refer to this type of situation as hereditary predisposition. So, within an individual cell there may be a hereditary predisposition to cancer.

As well as this, either in combination or independently, the DNA can be influenced by external chemical stimuli which can lead to the haphazard and uncontrolled cellular division which is the characteristic hallmark of cancer. These external stimuli include, among others, viruses, hormones, harmful chemicals and ionizing radiation.

Can viruses cause cancer?

There has always been a school of scientific thought that has strongly believed that the basic cause of many cancers can be attributed to viral infection. But, while there are well-documented cases of viruses causing cancer in animals, there is, on the whole, little evidence for this in humans. However, specifically, there are three rare cancers which are almost certainly caused by viruses. These are 'human T-cell leukaemia', Burkitt's lymphoma (see page 115), and nasopharyngeal carcinoma. Similarly, viral particles have been isolated in cancers of the breast and liver though the significance of such particles is still very much open to debate.

One of the major problems when considering whether or not viruses are a cause of cancer is the fact that when they enter body tissues, viruses tend to set up an inflammatory reaction. This inflammatory reaction can then become chronic and it is possible that if the cells of the involved tissues become cancerous, the malignancy may be due to chronic inflammation, rather than from the viral particles themselves.

Can the AIDS virus cause cancer?

This question is extremely important because it throws up a basic concept which I believe probably underlies some of the causes of the various cancers.

Let us recall what happens in cancer. I explained earlier that the normal cells begin dividing in an abnormal way and that their division remains unchecked, allowing them to grow out of control. The internal control mechanisms of the cancer cells appear, therefore, to have broken down or have been circumvented. But this is not the end of the story.

The body has a secondary defence mechanism to cope with cells that are growing out of control. This mechanism is known as the immune system. You may have come across this term and may associate it with infections – especially bacterial infections – and indeed the immune system *is* responsible for combating both bacterial and viral infections. But it has another role, that of keeping a close surveillance on all the tissues of the body. If it notices that certain cells look as though they are liable to grow out of control and become cancerous, the immune system removes them.

The immune system works in the following manner. It is composed of cells known as white cells and blood proteins known as antibodies. These white cells and antibodies gain access to most parts of the body via the bloodstream, where they are predominantly found, although they are produced in the bone marrow and in the lymph nodes (see p.115).

The AIDS virus prevents the body's immune system from functioning effectively. This breakdown results in two problems. Firstly, normally mild infections can get out of hand and sweep through the AIDS sufferer's body. Secondly, the immune system fails to detect and pick out those cells which are dividing abnormally (i.e., cancer cells). More recently it has been proposed that the problem may not lie entirely within the immune system. But, rather, the cancerous cells are not recognized by a normally functioning immune system because, on their surfaces, they do not possess what is known as a normal 'chemical marker' (antigen) that allows them to be recognized by the immune system.

So, it seems that from this terrible disease, AIDS, we might at least learn and eventually be able to treat what is possibly the fundamental problem in the causation of cancer: the breakdown of the body's immune system with the consequent eruption of cancerous growths. In general terms, what AIDS teaches us is that if the body's immune system is somehow damaged, cancerous cells can remain undetected.

Can chemicals cause cancer?

Chemicals can definitely cause cancer and it is important that we talk about those that may do so because it is obviously important that they should be identified and avoided. This is an example of an all-important principle with cancer, and many other diseases: prevention.

The best example of a cancer that is caused by a chemical is lung cancer, which is heavily linked to smoking. The precise nature of the chemical that causes lung cancer has not as yet been identified but it is felt that one of the many chemicals that are found in cigarette tar is almost certainly responsible.

Another chemical which may play a part in lung cancer is blue asbestos, once used extensively to insulate heating systems. This can cause a particularly rare form of lung cancer known as mesothelioma (see p.76). Lung cancer may also be caused by chromium and nickel, these cancers being restricted mainly to those who work in industries involving particular substances. Other examples of 'industrial' cancers have been found in the nasal sinuses of some woodworkers and in the livers of workers in certain plastics industries.

These are but a few examples of chemicals that can cause cancer. But if you happen to work in industries which use any of these chemicals, do not worry unduly about the risk of developing cancer. Not only is the risk small, but, now that we are alerted to the possibility of cancers being caused by certain industrial processes, there is a very high level of monitoring of all such processes so that the risks of contracting cancer at your place of work are now almost negligible.

Can certain foods cause cancer?

Some chemicals taken in the diet have been shown to promote cancer. In some cereal crops, such as maize, that are stored under unsatisfactory conditions, certain moulds can produce chemical substances called aflatoxins which have been found to have a direct link with liver cancer. This has particularly been found to be the case in certain African countries.

Much attention has been given lately to the effects of nitrates in our diet. Nitrates are used as fertilizers and are ingested on fresh vegetables. In the body they are converted to chemicals known as nitrosamines which, under experimental conditions, have been shown to be cancer-forming, though there does not appear to be any clear link between nitrates and human cancer.

There is also concern over many of the artificial sweeteners and additives that are used in food and drinks which are part and parcel of our modern way of living. For example, cyclamate – a synthetic sweetener – has been shown to cause cancer in animals, as have various antioxidants and similar additives. I must emphasize, however, that none of these has been shown to cause cancer in human beings. Indeed, certain food additives that are preservative probably result in a reduced incidence of cancer.

Medical dietary opinion is pointing towards the possibility that certain cancers – in particular those of the stomach and bowel – may be caused by dietary factors but as yet there is little concrete evidence for this assumption.

Can ultraviolet light cause skin cancer?

Ultraviolet light is a form of radiation. It is found in natural light and is that part of sunlight that is responsible for tanning our skins. If unprotected skin is overexposed to ultraviolet light, there is a possibility that it may develop skin cancer. This problem is most commonly seen in fair-skinned people who either spend a lot of time outdoors, in bright sunlight, or who live in permanently sunny climates as in Australia.

It has recently become fashionable to have tanning treatments on sunbeds. Whether or not the levels of ultraviolet radiation that people receive on sunbeds is in the long term going to produce a crop of skin cancers only time will tell, but I would strongly advise you to be very careful when exposing yourself to ultraviolet radiation in this way.

But ultraviolet light is not the only form of radiation that can give you cancer.

What other forms of radiation can cause cancer?

The association between radioactivity and cancer is well known as seen in the survivors of the atomic bombs at Nagasaki and Hiroshima. But there are many forms of radiation.

One radioactive compound, for example, is widely distributed in the earth. This compound is radium, and it gives off a radioactive gas called radon. Although radon levels are extremely low, it is believed that this 'background radiation' can cause cancers, especially those affecting blood, called leukaemias.

Many people worry about radioactive levels in X-rays and are concerned that X-rays may do them harm, even causing them cancer. It is true that in the past X-rays did cause cancer. Now that the danger has been realized, however, the problem has been eliminated.

Such patients should not worry. The amount of radiation now given in X-rays – even in a fairly extensive course – falls far short of the dosages that can cause cancer.

Can cancer be inherited?

Only in exceptional circumstances and with very rare forms of cancer. In the vast majority of cases there is no real evidence to suggest that cancer can be inherited. Statistical assessments on the subject have been so exhaustive that I believe this to be, in general terms, a fair and accurate statement.

That being so, however, the case for cancer *not* being an inherited disease is not completely proven. It has been shown, for example, that the risk of developing breast cancer is higher in female relatives of women who already have the disease than in the rest of the female population as a whole. Though, as we shall see, this may be due to environmental rather than genetic factors.

There is a rather nebulous concept of 'cancer families' in which it appears that the likelihood of cancer arising in members of particular families is higher than in others. I must emphasize that there is no hard statistical evidence to support this idea, however, and that the term 'cancer families' should therefore be avoided.

Finally, some rare forms of cancers *can* be inherited. One is a cancer of the eye known as retinoblastoma; another is a skin condition called xeroderm pigmentosa. Such cancers are extremely rare, however, and have only been mentioned here as exceptions.

Can hormones cause cancer?

Hormones are proteins that are produced by a variety of special glands in the body, known as endocrine glands. They are secreted into and carried by the blood to their destinations, known as target organs. There is no real evidence to suggest that hormones initiate the cancer process but there is no doubt that in certain circumstances, when a cancer is either establishing itself or is rapidly increasing in size, they can encourage the cancerous cells to grow at a greater rate.

Such cancers are referred to as being 'hormone-dependent'. Some forms of breast cancer (see p.54) are hormone dependent, the hormone in question being oestrogen.

In the cancer of the male prostate gland (see p.107), however, an artificially manufactured drug called stilboestrol, which is chemically similar to the hormone oestrogen, can actually cause a regression of prostatic cancer – an example of how, in certain cases, hormones can *beneficially* influence the growth of cancerous tissue.

In pregnancy, existing cancers of the breast and cervix (see pp.52, 91) can be worsened due to certain hormonal levels that accompany pregnancy.

However, metastatic, or secondary, spread has sometimes been seen to regress during the course of a pregnancy.

Can cancer develop as a by-product of chronic non-cancerous disease?

Chronic diseases are so called because they often take a long time to appear and, once established, are very difficult to eradicate. An example of such a problem is the varicose ulcers that can form in the skin of legs affected by varicose veins. Sometimes, when the margins of these ulcers are carefully examined under a microscope they can show signs of early cancerous changes next to the area of chronic inflammation. Similarly, in ulcerative colitis of the large bowel, in which there is a chronic inflammation of the bowel wall, small areas of bowel cancer can break out amidst the areas of general chronic inflammation. Chronic inflammation can also be found in the liver – a problem known as cirrhosis of the liver. In nine out of ten cases where cancer arises in the liver it will be found to be superimposed on cirrhosis of the liver.

In more general terms, there is a condition called 'the precancerous lesion'. This refers to a specific area or tissue of the body that, although not demonstrating obvious cancerous change, will go on to develop cancer in the future. It is important to be aware of this concept of the precancerous state, for if the problem can be spotted and treated early, cancer will not develop. One example of the precancerous state is leucoplakia – a condition whereby little white areas can develop on the tongue or on the lining of the mouth of elderly people (not to be confused with the fungal condition popularly known as 'thrush' often found in infants).

Can drugs cause cancer?

All drugs are extensively tested and are only allowed on the market when it is absolutely certain that, among other things, they will not cause cancer. However, I would like to illustrate with one example how important it is that the medical profession remains alert to the possibility that drugs can cause cancer.

In the 1950s, in America, an oestrogen compound was routinely given to pregnant women who were threatening to miscarry. Many of these women did not miscarry and went on to produce what appeared to be quite normal babies. When these children grew up, however, it was discovered that some of the girls had developed a very rare form of cancer, cancer of the vagina, which was directly attributable to the oestrogen drug that their mothers had received in pregnancy.

Not only does this indicate how careful doctors must be before prescribing any drug, especially during pregnancy, it also demonstrates that there can be a long latent period before a cancer can develop which can sometimes make it very difficult to identify the actual initiating cause of the cancer.

Can psychological factors cause cancer?

This is a question that has been asked for centuries. As far back as AD 200 the Greek philosopher and physician Galen suggested that 'melancholy' women were more susceptible to breast cancer. Much later, in the eighteenth century, the physician Gendron suggested that both stress and depression were causes of cancer. In the nineteenth century another doctor, Walshe, reported that those of his patients who had depressive features were more prone to the disease. More recently, when psychologists have assessed certain groups of cancer patients, they have demonstrated psychological factors which, they claim, have a bearing on the development of cancer.

Whatever the significance of these findings and suggestions, they reinforce what is an important concept: a multifactorial cause of cancer.

Psychological factors are known to have a direct influence on many of the body's physiological functions. Additionally, physiological functions exhibit a delicate balance between each other. To see how complex these interactions can be, let's draw together some facts that we have already discussed and consider how they relate to this balance between the body's physiological and psychological components.

When I was talking about the basic causes of cancer, I mentioned that one of the basic faults lay in the body's immune system and its failure to detect and eliminate cancer cells, or that cancer cells somehow avoid being detected by the immune system. But the immune system does not work on its own, in isolation; it can be influenced by both psychological and physiological factors. It can also be influenced by the central nervous system as well as the endocrine system, which is responsible for hormonal secretion. Consequently, the immune system can be functionally depressed by changes in the body's hormonal status or by the influence of the brain.

Both these physiological systems may in turn be directly influenced by an individual's psychological status. Factors such as stress or depression may cause changes both in the hormonal and immune systems which, as we have seen, may influence the growth of cancers.

Some cancers can arise in areas of chronic inflammation. An example of this is ulcerative colitis, a chronic inflammatory condition of the large bowel. Ulcerative colitis itself is, in certain circumstances, a recognized manifestation of underlying psychological problems. Thus, although psychological factors cannot be said to be directly responsible for the bowel cancer that sometimes develops in individuals with ulcerative colitis, they probably play a supporting role.

A much more direct example of how psychological factors may exert an influence on the development of cancer can be seen in the well-known association between cigarette-smoking and lung cancer. Many people smoke cigarettes because they find the sensation reduces stress, though, by smoking, they will probably increase the chances of contracting lung cancer (or heart disease).

So, from this brief look at the influence of psychological factors on cancer, you can see that factors such as stress and depression probably exert many different and subtle effects. The complex integration of the central nervous system, the immune system and the endocrine system with their interdependence upon each other suggests that a person's psychological status may indeed have a bearing on the development of cancerous change. Whether or not people with particular types of personality are more likely to develop cancer, however, remains open to question.

If I am told that I have a tumour does it mean that I have cancer?

The precise meaning of words is of fundamental importance. Unless we get our definitions correct in the sense that we are all talking about the same thing, any amount of confusion can arise. It is all a question of good doctor–patient communication. Once terminology is bandied about, without proper explanation, misconceptions and misunderstandings arise.

The word 'tumour' is a good example of how this can happen. Tumours are commonly believed to be synonymous with cancer but medically this is not the case. Pathologically, the word 'tumour' embraces two major sub-divisions of tissue change: benign and malignant. Benign tumours are non-cancerous. Malignant tumours are cancerous.

Here is an example of how the use of the word 'tumour' can be confusing. In the uterus (womb) of a woman, muscular tissue can in certain areas grow excessively. These areas can be seen as swellings on the surface of the uterus and are called fibroids. Sometimes, when the nature of fibroids is being explained to a patient, the word 'tumour' is used to describe the fibroid. In the strict, technical sense, of course, a fibroid *is* a tumour, but it is a *benign tumour*, a *non-cancerous* tumour.

This is a typical situation where a patient may misunderstand what her doctor has told her and automatically assumes that she has cancer. She may feel that her doctor, by using the term tumour is, in some way, gently breaking the news that she has cancer. If, therefore, when you are consulting your doctor, the word tumour is mentioned, be sure to ask specifically whether the tumour is cancerous.

While on this subject of definitions I would like to mention a few other words that tend to crop up when cancer and cancer-related subjects are talked about.

One such term is 'neoplasia'. This is used to describe tissue that is demonstrating new, additional growth. In some cases this growth can be benign (non-cancerous), but in others it can be malignant (cancerous). Sometimes the world 'carcinoma ' is used instead of cancer. Carcinoma refers to a particular form of cancer arising from certain cells that line organs or areas of tissue. 'Mitotic lesion' is another way in which a cancerous growth is described. Broad terms such as 'swelling', 'collection of fluid', 'ulcer', 'spot' and 'lesion' should not be used. They are vague, and if they *are* used, be sure to ask your doctor to be more precise.

Finally, a word of warning about misinterpretation of what is being said. You will probably at some time in your life be admitted to hospital for either an operation or routine investigations. During your hospital stay, you will be visited by your consultant together with his entourage which may include medical students and student nurses. Often, on ward rounds, as well as dealing with specific patient problems, there is an element of discussion and teaching, and it is not uncommon for the medical staff, whilst grouped around a bed, to be discussing a topic that has nothing to do with your particular problem. In such circumstances, you may catch a word which you may recognize as having a cancerous association (perhaps one of the words which we have just been discussing).

If you feel that your doctors are discussing your particular case, with cancer in mind, ask them directly if what they were talking about was referring directly to you. Over the years, I have come across many patients who have worried unnecessarily, having picked up a chance remark made not about themselves but about another patient. If you are in any doubt, therefore, ask your doctor precisely what he means.

Can where I live be related to cancer?

The study of populations and disease is called epidemiology.

In the case of cancer, epidemiology has been an invaluable tool. A significant example of its success was the demonstration in the 1950s and 1960s by Sir Richard Doll that smoking could be directly related to lung cancer and, moreover, was the principal cause of the disease.

Other epidemiological surveys have shown some fascinating geographical characteristics. For instance, in studies of stomach cancer in the UK, it can be shown that the incidence of this disease is highest in North

Wales and the Fen district of Norfolk and Lincolnshire. Why this is so is not entirely clear though some have suggested that it may be due to the high peat content of the soil in these areas.

Epidemiological studies of other racial groupings have revealed many other interesting facts. They have shown, for example, that while cancer of the stomach is common amongst the Japanese, the incidence of the disease amongst those Japanese who have moved away from Japan and are living in the USA is exactly the same as in the general American population. It has been suggested that the reason for this is not, as was first thought, that Japanese people are racially particularly susceptible to stomach cancer but, rather, that there is something in their diet in Japan that may cause the disease. Similar interesting epidemiological surveys have shown that bowel cancer is much more common in Western than in African countries, though, once again, when Africans, as a group, move to the USA they demonstrate the same incidence of cancer of the bowel as does the general American population. Once again, diet is implicated. The main difference between the African and Western diet is that the African diet is considerably higher in fibre. It has been suggested that the reason why Westerners are so much more prone to bowel cancer is because of the slow passage of their food through their bowels due to its low fibre content. As a consequence, carcinogens (cancer-inducing substances) in the faeces stay in the large bowel for a longer time, causing the lining cells of the bowel to become cancerous.

Cancer of the oesophagus has been shown to be more common in Africans living around the shores of Lake Victoria. Again, this does not seem to be a racial predisposition but, rather, is due to a carcinogen in the maize which is used in the production of certain local drinks.

Recently, in Cumbria, epidemiological surveys on the local population have suggested that excessive amounts of radiation have contributed to an increase of cancers, especially in children (though, at the present time, there does not appear to be any statistical evidence to support this).

So, on the face of it, although where you live can be related to particular forms of cancer, just because you are of a particular race or live in a particular area does not necessarily mean that you will contract the disease.

Are certain age groups prone to particular types of cancer?

Although the incidence of cancer is relatively low in children it is never-theless responsible for an increasing proportion of serious illness in this age group, particularly in the form of leukaemia and brain tumours. In young people, as well as leukaemia, other less common forms of cancer may be seen which include a bone tumour called osteosarcoma as well as tumours of the lymph nodes known as lymphomas. In these younger age groups, cancer of the lung and of the bowel and other common cancers seen in the mature adult are almost unknown. In middle and early old age the common cancers predominate. Interestingly, in those over the age of 80, the incidence of malignancy decreases slightly though the reason for this is not known.

What types of cancer are there?

There are as many types of cancers as there are tissues in the body. But although almost every tissue in the body can undergo cancerous change, the most common sites of cancer are the lung, cervix, breast and bowel. There is always a problem with specific cancer descriptions, however, because different sorts of cancers can arise in the same structure or tissue.

Let's take cancer of the lung as an example. Cancerous tissue can arise in the lining cells of the bronchi (air passages), which permeate the lung tissue. This form of lung cancer is known as carcinoma of the bronchus. Earlier, when discussing the various causes of cancer I mentioned that asbestos can cause a particular form of lung cancer called mesothelioma.

This form of cancer is quite distinct from carcinoma of the bronchus, however, since it develops in the pleura (outer lining) of the lung.

So medically, rather than classifying cancers according to the particular organs that they affect, a more precise method is to describe them in terms of the particular types of tissue in which they arise. Following this classification, therefore, cancers can be divided into three groups: carcinomas, sarcomas and leukaemias. Carcinomas are cancerous changes in tissues that cover or line body organs; for instance, the lining cells of the bronchus, bowel or bladder, known as epithelial cells. Carcinomas can also develop in tissues that secrete various substances such as hormones; for example, the pancreas and the breast.

Sarcomas are cancers which arise in connective tissues such as nerve, muscle and bone. Certain brain tumours are examples of sarcomas.

Leukaemias most commonly refer to cancers of the blood cells and the cells of the immune system that are found in the lymph nodes.

I have mentioned this classification simply because you may come across it in other books or hear your doctor talk about it. In general terms, however, it is still much easier to think of cancer as arising in a particular organ rather than having to relate it to this rather more complicated concept.

What are the most common cancers?

The most common cancers are cancers of the lung, breast, uterus, prostate and bowel. Cancers of the bladder, stomach and the leukaemias are also relatively common. However, there are two important facts to remember here. Firstly, as we have just discussed, a lot can depend on where you live and how old you are. Secondly, the incidence of some cancers is not constant. For instance, the incidence of stomach cancer is going down while the rate of lung cancer is going up; the incidence of breast cancer remains about the same while those of cervical and uterine cancer are falling.

Are certain cancers more common in men than women?

Statistics show that certain cancers are more common in men than women once cancer of the breast, uterus and prostate have been removed from the figures. For example, lung cancer is more common in men than in women, though the incidence of lung cancer in women is rising. Similarly, cancers of the bladder are twice as common in men than in women. On the other hand, cancer of the gallbladder and the thyroid gland are more common in women than in men.

When looking at the differences between the sexes as regards the incidence not only of cancer but of other diseases, it is important to remember that women live longer than men. This means that these figures are almost certainly clouded by the fact that many men die of heart and vascular problems at an earlier age.

Had these men lived it is possible that they might well have developed cancers and so the figures would be changed.

Can cancers spread in the body?

Yes, cancer can spread from one part of the body to another. The initiating cancer is called the 'primary' cancer and the cancer that has spread is called the 'secondary' cancer. If the secondary cancer spreads to a distant part of the body it is called a metastasis, the spread itself being referred to as metastatic.

Cancers can spread in a number of different ways. Sometimes they spread within the area in which they first occur and this is termed a 'local' spread, as, for example, when breast cancer spreads locally within the breast.

At other times they can be spread by the bloodstream. Most tumours, at some stage, come into contact with blood vessels. If they erode the walls of these blood vessels some of the tumorous cells will enter the blood and they are then spread by the bloodstream to various parts of the body.

There is also another series of channels in the body that allows for communication between various tissues, and this is known as the lymphatic system. The lymphatic vessels are much more delicate than blood vessels but nevertheless, just like the bloodstream, they can take certain cancer cells from one part of the body to another.

The most common places for the secondary cancers to come to rest are in the bones, in the liver, the lungs and the brain. Sometimes it is due to these secondary cancerous deposits that the primary cancers come to be discovered, though by the time the cancer has spread it is usually at an advanced stage.

Can cancer be transmitted from one person to another?

Cancer is not an infectious disease and there is no evidence that cancer can be transmitted from one person to another. In my earlier discussion on AIDS (see p.10) I mentioned that the cause of this disease was a virus and that this virus could, indirectly, by affecting the immune system, cause cancer. It is only in this indirect way that cancer can be transmitted from one individual to another, and AIDS is probably the only example of this phenomenon.

General Clinical Aspects

What are common symptoms of cancer?

As I have already emphasized, many symptoms that are associated with cancer are also associated with other diseases. It is important, therefore, as you read these pages, that you do not immediately assume that you have cancer just because one or more of the symptoms that I describe happen to closely resemble a particular symptom of your own. There are many diseases that can affect the human body but the symptoms by which these diseases manifest themselves are few. If you are in any doubt as to your own symptoms seek the advice of your doctor. Doctors are only too glad to reassure any patient whose symptom is of no consequence, rather than have to confirm an advanced diagnosis of cancer. Remember, if you *do* have cancer, early diagnosis and treatment will greatly improve your overall long-term well-being. In the following pages I shall describe some of the common symptoms that can be indicative of cancer but at the same time I will also show how such symptoms can easily be caused by non-cancerous diseases. I hope that this will serve two purposes: it will show how some trivial symptom should not be ignored but will also demonstrate that such symptoms are not necessarily cancerous in origin.

Does cancer cause pain?

It is a common misconception that cancer automatically causes pain. Many cancers, even in their advanced stages, do not cause pain. The first important point to emphasize is that just because you have cancer it does not necessarily mean to say that you will inevitably experience pain. Pain does accompany some cancers, but with modern techniques and therapies such pain can be controlled (see pp. 139-141).

Should I be worried if I find a lump or lumps in or under my skin, especially in or around my breasts? Is this a sure sign of cancer?

All lumps that appear in the skin should be taken seriously and any lump that appears in the breast should be taken extremely seriously. Having said that, although such lumps can, indeed, be cancerous it is far more likely that they are simply benign swellings. Breast lumps and breast cancer will be discussed more fully on pp.52-75, but here I should like to mention benign breast lumps and swellings. Even though a lump may appear out of the blue and even though it may appear to be hard (one of the characteristics of a cancerous growth), it is much more likely to be a benign tumour termed a fibroadenoma. This is an example of a symptom that could be cancer but which is more likely to be a benign problem.

Other examples can be found in the armpits and groins, where there are collections of lymph nodes, an integral part of the body's immune system. When these lymph nodes are active, they can swell and be felt just beneath the surface of the skin. Like breast lumps, they should receive immediate medical advice but again, in the vast majority of cases, they will turn out to be the body's response to an infection rather than cancer. So, although any lumps which appear should be taken seriously, the vast majority will prove to be benign.

Can ulcers and skin blemishes be cancer?

Ulcers on superficial surfaces of the body can naturally occur in or around the mouth and nose, on the genital organs or around the ankles. Ulcers in and around the mouth and nose are almost always due to a viral infection, while on the genitals they are often due to a sexually transmitted disease. Ulcers around the ankle are normally due to poor circulation and even though they may be taking time to heal it does not follow that they are cancerous.

Blemishes on the skin which are long standing are almost certainly not cancerous. If, however, you notice a blemish that has newly appeared, or seems to be growing, changing shape or colour, is itchy or bleeds intermittently, then this should receive medical attention for while these signs may be the result of a harmless skin condition, they may also be symptoms of early skin cancer (see pp.104-106).

Can a change in my appetite or bowel habits be indicative of cancer?

Loss of appetite, loss of weight, feelings of discomfort in the upper abdomen and intermittent abdominal pain following meals must always be taken seriously. These symptoms will usually be due to either a benign stomach or duodenal ulcer, gallbladder disease, a problem with food absorption, or simply, stress. However, they may be indicative of early stomach or bowel cancer and it is therefore essential that you seek medical advice.

Other symptoms to watch out for are a change in bowel habit – either constipation or diarrhoea – and blood in faeces. More often than not the change in bowel habit will be caused by a change in diet, and the bleeding due to haemorrhoids (piles), but such symptoms can be indicative of cancerous growth and your doctor's advice should be sought.

Should I go to my doctor if I find that my urine is discoloured?

It is often difficult by just looking at the colour of urine to decide whether or not there is blood or some other substance in it. Urine can show different colours at different times. If you notice that the colour of your urine is different than usual, this symptom should be taken seriously, especially if the urine contains obvious traces of blood. Such a symptom is probably due to an infection of the urinary system, but it can be indicative of cancer of the bladder.

To illustrate how such symptoms can give undue worry, blood in the urine can sometimes be seen in male joggers. The reasons for this are unclear and the problem harmless but such bleeding should nevertheless always be fully investigated.

Can a chronic cough or hoarseness mean that I have cancer?

Coughs are common in people who smoke; cancer is common in people who smoke. These facts inevitably pose a problem.

Smoking tends to cause chronic bronchitis, the characteristic features of which are chronic coughing together with the bringing up of phlegm (spit/sputum). It is often said that a persistent cough can be a sign of cancer.

This is certainly the case and the cause of the cough should be thoroughly investigated. But many bronchitics cough their way through life. Some never develop cancer whereas others eventually do. This obviously poses a diagnostic problem. How often should such people attend their doctors? How often should they be thoroughly investigated? The simple solution to the problem is, clearly, to give up smoking. If you are a smoker with chronic bronchitis and you notice that your cough is becoming more persistent, and especially if your spit contains traces of blood, then it is essential that you tell your doctor. For non-smokers with a cough that appears to be persistent, following influenza or a chest infection, the likelihood that this is due to cancer is extremely remote but, again, such symptoms should not be ignored.

Hoarseness may sometimes accompany chronic bronchitis, especially when there has been excessive coughing. In somebody who does not smoke it is a symptom that must be taken seriously. In the majority of cases it will be due to laryngitis or, surprisingly, a deficiency of thyroid hormone, but, very rarely, it may be due to cancer of the larynx (voice box).

If my periods are irregular or if I have bleeding between periods is this a symptom of cancer?

Irregular menstrual bleeding in young women is rarely due to cancer.

In older women who are premenopausal, such irregular bleeding can be due to a number of benign conditions such as non-cancerous swellings of the uterus (womb), called fibroids, or benign growths (polyps).

However, in both these groups of women, both cervical cancer and uterine cancer can present as irregular bleeding or as an abnormal vaginal discharge.

One answer to this problem is cervical screening. But even though you have had cervical screening and you notice such symptoms then it is advisable that you go to your doctor for a repeat cervical check and examination.

In older women, following the menopause, any vaginal bleeding must be taken very seriously, and immediately reported to your doctor. He will almost certainly refer you to a consultant gynaecologist but even if this happens do not worry. Cancer of the uterus is a possibility but there are many other possibilities. Although you will be investigated to exclude the diagnosis of cancer do not assume that just because you have this symptom you have cancer.

Remember, ask your doctor at every stage of the investigations if he has anything positive to report.

Are there any more general symptoms of cancer that I should be aware of?

There are many general symptoms that can be due to cancer but I must yet again emphasize that these can also be caused by many other conditions. In fact, cancer is rarely diagnosed from symptoms alone. The symptoms will merely alert both you and your doctor to the possibility that something is wrong. Many of the diagnostic investigations that you will undergo will nevertheless be directed at excluding cancer.

It is sometimes worrying when you go to your doctor with vague symptoms to find yourself the subject of a battery of investigations. You may feel that these will inevitably lead to a diagnosis of cancer. But try not to worry if you find yourself investigated in this way. The purpose of these tests is as much to exclude a diagnosis of cancer as to confirm one.

One of the general features that can characterize cancer is weight loss but there are many other conditions in which weight loss features as a presenting symptom. These include psychological causes such as stress or anxiety, changes in dietary habit or an inability of the body to absorb food. Sometimes, too, weight loss can be due to a gastric or duodenal ulcer, or disease of the liver, gallbladder or pancreas.

Another general feature of cancer is that of feeling 'below par', a feeling known medically as lassitude, the sort of feeling that you can often get following recovery from a severe bout of 'flu. Once again, however, countless diseases – both psychological and physical – can account for these nebulous symptoms.

A word here about pain. Because cancer is commonly associated with pain it is often assumed that painful symptoms may be cancerous in origin. In fact, pain is normally a late symptom of cancer, and with many cancers there is no element of pain at all. I mentioned earlier that some cancers can spread to other parts of the body. When these cancers (known as metastases or 'secondaries') lodge in bone, they can cause pain. When they arise in the bones of the spinal column, they can cause collapse of these bones together with consequent entrapment of the nerves which are passing through them. This problem is known as vertebral collapse.

If you are experiencing pain anywhere in your body, therefore, go and have it checked out, although the likelihood of it being cancerous in origin is slight.

When considering the common symptoms of cancer, it is apparent that in many cases the symptom can rarely be said to be a specific symptom of a particular type of cancer. Some symptoms are trivial and remain so. Other symptoms appear trivial but may eventually lead to a diagnosis of cancer. The message, therefore, is this. If you have a symptom that is worrying you, *go and see your doctor*. Remember, doctors would far rather spend a little time diagnosing a trivial complaint than have to confront you with a diagnosis of cancer that may be at an advanced stage. Do not ignore your symptoms, especially if they are symptoms that you do not normally have.

What should I do if I think I have cancer?

If you have reason to think that you might have cancer you must go and see your general practitioner. More often than not what you have will be a passing problem but it may be the first hint of cancer. If so, your chances will be vastly improved by an early diagnosis.

Alternatively, you may have gone to your general practitioner with what you considered to be a trivial problem and during the course of the conversation and examination he openly raises the possibility of cancer or, in passing, mentions that there is a possibility of cancer.

Similarly, the tests that he has arranged for you might well start your mind ticking over to the possibility that your doctor thinks you have cancer (this may well, in fact, be why you are reading this book).

If such thoughts are worrying you do not bottle them up, but ask your doctor directly if he thinks that you might have cancer. Once more, I cannot emphasize too strongly that cancer is potentially a serious problem and that it is always important for your doctor to begin by excluding the possibility that you have it.

When you go to your doctor with a specific symptom he will probably ask you a few simple questions. These will include the length of time that you have had the symptoms, whether or not they are constant, and whether they come and go.

He will also probably ask if you have noticed any particular change in bodily habits, such as appetite, bowel function, weight (both gain and loss), sleeping patterns and whether you have experienced spikes of temperature or abnormal periods of excessive sweating. The list is enormous. Suffice to say that we all know what we are like normally and can recognize when our bodies are not behaving normally.

Before going to your doctor you may find it particularly helpful to jot down your symptoms and as many details about your abnormal bodily functions as possible. This will be helpful in two ways. Firstly, it will help your doctor to form a much more accurate picture of your symptoms and, secondly, it will help you to remember to give your doctor all the details about the problem. We all know how easy it is to forget essential things when we are nervous and worried.

When you have finished explaining the nature of the problem to your doctor he will then probably ask you a few more questions, including whether there is a family history of cancer. Just because he asks you this do not jump immediately to the conclusion that he, therefore, automatically assumes that you have cancer. He is simply looking for an overall picture of your medical background and, naturally, your family medical history is of importance.

The doctor will then examine you, concentrating on the particular part of your anatomy that appears to be causing you problems. Having completed his examination he may well then arrange for you to have some tests.

What tests will my GP do?

It is not generally appreciated, but one of the less heralded revolutions in medicine has occurred in primary health care. This is the availability to GPs of many investigatory facilities which, in the past, could only be used by a specialist consultant at the hospital. This more readily available access benefits the patient because a GP can instigate the tests right away, using valuable time that was formerly lost waiting for a hospital appointment. It also reduces the burden on the hospital consultant who finds himself with more time to deal with the problems that the GP's investigations have thrown up.

In later chapters I shall look at the individual tests carried out for specific cancers but in general terms, the following are normally routine investigations.

First your doctor will take a blood test. Much can be learned about bodily functions from this. It will establish whether or not you are anaemic, how your liver, kidneys (and, to some extent, pancreas) are functioning. It can also give valuable information about your hormones, and in some cases may actually show direct chemical evidence of cancer.

Your GP may well then ask you for specimens of sputum or urine. If you are a woman and have not had a cervical smear this will be done.

These specimens are then sent to the cytology laboratory where direct evidence of cancer cells will be looked for.

There is also a host of X-ray investigations that your doctor can directly request.

He will normally do this by writing out his request on an X-ray form which you yourself then take up to the hospital to the radiology department. Such investigations commonly include X-rays of the chest, of the skull, various bones and the abdomen. He will also be able to request special X-rays of your kidneys (see pp.34, 125) and special investigations of your digestive system (see pp.101-102). Having all this spadework done by the GP will, in many cases, alleviate the fear of having to go to hospital to see an unfamiliar doctor, and undergoing a battery of strange tests.

By the time your GP has carried out these initial tests he will be in a position to tell you one of two things: that his tests have thrown up the cause of your symptoms and that there is no need for any further investigations, or that some of the results need further investigation and a consultant opinion. Even at this stage, however, do not automatically feel that just because you are going to see a consultant this necessarily means there is something seriously wrong with you. The problem may simply have arisen because of ambiguities in some of your test results and more specialized tests will be needed in order to arrive at a definite diagnosis.

So, don't jump to conclusions. If you are worried, always ask direct questions.

What happens when I am referred to a consultant?

Your consultant, like your GP, is a doctor, the only difference being that he has a specialist knowledge in a particular field of medicine. He will also have access, if needs be, to more detailed and more specific tests that will lead to a definite diagnosis of your condition. In addition, he will be an expert in the treatment of your particular problem and will be able to initiate the treatment and carry it out with the co-operation of your GP. When you go up to the hospital to see your consultant for the first time, not only will he have in front of him a detailed referral letter from your GP, he may also have the results of any tests your GP has already carried out. By the time you get to see him, therefore, he will already have a very good idea of the problem he is dealing with. Nevertheless, he will go over your symptoms again with you to make sure that nothing has been overlooked. He will also give you a thorough medical examination. On the basis of the information supplied to him by the GP, he may then do one of two things. If the GP's test results are ambiguous, he will probably ask for these to be repeated and will ask to see you again in a matter of one or two weeks when these results are back. On the other hand, he may feel, from what he already knows, that further, more specialized, tests should be carried out. Even though these tests might be more specialized, some can be done on an outpatient basis, though others may require a brief hospital stay. If you are asked to go into hospital for your tests, therefore, do not panic. Once again, this doesn't necessarily mean that you have got anything seriously wrong with you. It just means that it would be easier for you and your doctors to perform the investigations in hospital rather than on an outpatient basis.

What is likely to happen to me when I am called into hospital for tests

On pp.52-129 I shall be going more fully into the specific types of tests carried out for each cancer. Here I shall simply mention, in general terms, some of the tests you may come across, though you will certainly not be subjected to all of them.

First, a few words about what is entailed in being admitted to hospital for routine tests. Later in the book I shall be discussing the procedures for a specific admission to hospital for surgery to remove a cancer, but there is a great difference between being admitted to hospital for a formal operation and being admitted for tests. In the latter case, you are not ill in the acute sense of the word and will find that the nursing staff will treat you accordingly. You will not, for example, normally be asked to undress and get into bed.

The first doctor you will come across will be the houseman, or junior doctor on your consultant's medical team. He will formally admit you, which will involve him asking you questions that you have probably already been asked before and carrying out an examination that will almost certainly have been done by both your GP and your consultant. Don't worry that things are being duplicated in this way. It is just possible that he may find something that both your GP and your consultant have overlooked. These multiple checks help to eliminate mistakes that can inevitably creep into any organization.

Following this you will probably be seen by your consultant. He will check that your admission has gone smoothly and that the tests that he ordered for you in the outpatients department are in hand. Once this is done the tests for which you have been admitted will then begin.

What sort of tests am I likely to have?

These tests can be divided into two groups. The first can be carried out either on the ward or in a theatre adjacent to the ward designed especially for this purpose. The second will take you off the ward and into the various specialist departments. This is normally because the apparatus for these tests cannot be brought to you. Don't worry that you will be put in a wheelchair and wheeled around the hospital like an invalid. You will normally be allowed to walk everywhere, though you may be accompanied by a nurse from the ward. After some of the tests, however, it may be advisable that you remain lying down for a certain length of time. Under these circumstances you may be taken back to the ward either in a chair or on a trolley.

Examples of ward tests are as follows. You will almost certainly have some blood tests. This is not simply a pointless repetition of the tests you have already had done.

The tests may well be the same, but, more importantly, the doctors will be looking for both confirmation of previous test results and any change in these results in order to see whether the tests show an improvement or a worsening of the situation.

There is also a test that is closely related to a blood test called a bone marrow biopsy. Since blood is manufactured in the bone marrow, it is a logical step to take a sample of this bone marrow and to examine it alongside the blood itself. The sample of bone marrow is usually taken from the iliac crest (hip bone). The procedure is slightly uncomfortable, any pain being deadened by a local anaesthetic.

You will see here that I have introduced the term biopsy. This is an important concept in terms of investigation. A biopsy is a sample piece of tissue taken from a particular area of the body. It is a small, representative area of tissue, which is examined under a microscope in the pathology laboratory and can indicate whether or not there is evidence of cancer in the tissue. Biopsies are taken in many different ways.

Biopsies of the pleura (lining of the lung), can be taken through the chest wall while liver biopsies are taken through the abdominal wall. All these procedures are conducted under local anaesthestic and, apart from minor discomfort, are generally painless and safe. Complete safety can never be guaranteed with any medical procedure, however, and this is one of the reasons for admitting you to hospital for investigation – so that, in the unlikely event of complications arising nurses and doctors will be on hand to cope immediately with any problems.

The next group of tests involve the use of fibre-optiscopes. These look rather like narrow garden hosepipes, and have the same flexible characteristics but, whereas the garden hosepipe carries water, the fibre-optiscope carries light. The particular property of the fibre-optiscope is that light can travel along it, even when it is bent. This allows examination of parts of the internal anatomy that are normally obscured from direct vision. By looking through the eye piece at one end of the fibre-optiscope your doctor can observe, for example, the lining of your stomach (gastroscopy, p.102) or the condition of your bronchial tree (bronchoscopy, p.80). In these situations, not only can your doctor have a good look at the internal aspects of the organ under investigation, but he can also, if he wishes, take a biopsy of tissue from any suspicious-looking areas. The results of such a biopsy will confirm or refute his previous clinical findings and will be of crucial importance for both diagnosis and treatment.

As I said before, these tests may be done on a ward or in a minor operating theatre. If it is the latter, don't worry. This doesn't mean that the tests will be either prolonged or complicated. The reasons for having to go to theatre are because specialized apparatus is often kept there, and the position that your body might have to be placed in to allow easy passage of instruments is often most easily achieved on modern versatile operating tables.

What sort of tests can I expect to undergo in the radiology department?

In the radiology, or X-ray department, the tests may well begin with similar X-rays to those that you have already had. Such repeat X-rays are routine and can help to establish whether or not there has been a change from previous X-rays.

Once these tests have been done you may then undergo what are known as 'contrast studies'. These involve introducing a radio-opaque material into the parts of your body that are under investigation, so that a particular organ can be highlighted, the radio-opaque material showing up on subsequent X-rays that are taken. Let's take a practical example to illustrate this. Let us assume that you have been having some upper abdominal discomfort. Your consultant may want to see whether or not the problem is due to a duodenal ulcer or stomach cancer. In the X-ray department you will be given a cupful of what looks like milk but which is in fact a barium compound.

Barium is entirely harmless when taken by mouth, but has the properties of being opaque when photographed by X-rays. You will be asked to drink the barium liquid and, as you do so, X-ray photographs will be taken as the barium liquid passes through your mouth, down your oesophagus (gullet) and into your stomach. The barium will then outline the upper part of your digestive tract, and a permanent record of any abnormalities or problems which this throws up can be kept on the X-rays for your consultant to see. Using the same principle a barium enema can be administered at the other end of the digestive tract. The state of the lower part of your digestive tract will thus be outlined in the same way and can then be examined for evidence of inflammation, polyps or cancer.

The gallbladder, which is an off-shoot of the digestive tract, can also be examined by contrast techniques. This time you will be given the contrast medium in capsules containing a dye. When you swallow the capsule, the dye is absorbed from the stomach, passes into the bloodstream and subsequently to the liver and gallbladder. X-ray photographs are then taken of the gallbladder, which is outlined by this contrast dye.

To examine the kidneys with the contrast dye technique, the dye actually has to be injected into your body via a vein in the arm. The kidneys will concentrate the dye from the bloodstream and will consequently be outlined. So too will be the tubes that join the kidneys to the bladder (known as the ureters). In this way the whole of the urinary tract can be observed. This procedure is known as an intravenous pyelogram (IVP). It is painless and poses no problems though you may experience a mild flushing sensation. You should, however, mention to the doctor who is giving you the injection if you have had any adverse reactions to IVPs in the past or if you are allergic to anything such as penicillin or other drugs.

I mentioned earlier that one of the ways that cancer can spread is by way of the lymph vessels which drain into lymph nodes. These lymph vessels, and their nodes, can be shown radiographically by injecting contrast dye into lymph vessels in the foot. The resulting X-rays will outline the fine ramifications of these vessels from the feet to the groins and into the abdomen.

Similarly, if a tumour is suspected in the region of the spinal column, contrast material can be injected into the fluid that surrounds the spinal cord. This fluid is known as the cerebro-spinal fluid and the technique is known as myelography.

Are there more modern radiological techniques than the ones you have described?

A third and separate type of X-ray investigation is now available known as the CAT scan or CT body scanning (the CT stands for computerized tomography). The marvellous thing about this machine is that it can, in photographic terms, 'slice' the body up into sections that look remarkably like internal anatomical pictures. CT scanning has revolutionized radiological diagnosis. Although it can, under certain circumstances, take quite a time to perform, it has managed to eliminate many of the other, more uncomfortable and now outdated, types of radiological tests.

What are liver scans and bone scans?

These involve administering a radioactive compound which settles in particular areas of disease in the body. Take, for example, a liver scan. Here, the radioactive compound is injected into the bloodstream and is taken up by the liver. If there is a tumour in the liver, the tumour, not being part of the normal liver tissue, will not take up the radioactive isotope. A special machine known as a gamma camera can take a 'picture' of the liver. The area of the liver that is affected by tumour will show up as a gap or a hole in the picture that the gamma camera produces.

Similar radioactive isotope scans can be made of the lungs, the kidneys and bone. They are used mostly to detect any areas of cancer spread.

What happens when these tests are completed?

Inevitably this period is worrying, for now you have to wait for the results of your tests. Rest assured that these will be given to you as soon as possible, though sometimes there are unavoidable delays. The results of the X-ray test will normally come through fairly quickly. Similarly, if you are having barium tests, the radiologist will actually be observing the progress of the investigation and will be able to see any signs of disease instantaneously. A phone call to your consultant means that such results can be communicated quickly.

However, sometimes the results from the radiology department may only narrow down the problem to a specific area of, say, the digestive tract and it is difficult to decide what is actually causing the problem. In such cases, biopsies must be taken of the actual tissue under investigation. And it is here that delays sometimes occur. The biopsy has to be processed in the pathology laboratory where it is prepared for examination. Preparation involves embedding the biopsy material in wax, cutting it into very thin sections, then staining it with specific chemical dyes so that its features may be seen more easily.

Once this is done the biopsy specimen is ready for mounting, and must then be looked at under the microscope by a consultant pathologist. All this takes time, which accounts for why there may sometimes be a delay in conveying the test results to your medical team.

The reason why it is so important that your own consultant gets the results of the biopsy is that he can not act without the biopsy result. It is one of the golden rules in treating a patient who might have cancer that no treatment is given until the biopsy result confirms that cancer is definitely present, what type of cancer it is and the stage (degree of malignancy) that it exhibits.

In most cases, once the tests are completed, you will be discharged from the hospital. The results of your tests will be communicated to you either by a member of the medical team that was looking after you in hospital or by your GP. He will be kept closely informed as to your progress and the results of your investigations either by letter or by telephone from the medical team at the hospital.

What happens if the tests show that I have cancer?

If the tests do show that you have cancer this information will normally be given to you by your consultant or sometimes by your GP. Your consultant will discuss with you the form of treatment he proposes to carry out. If you are given the news by your GP, however, he will be able to explain the outlines of the problem but will probably be unable to go any further, since it may be difficult for him to pre-judge what precise form of treatment your consultant will institute. He may, therefore, not be in a position to be definite about whether or not an operation will be necessary, and if so, what the operation will entail.

This time, between the definitive diagnosis and admission to hospital for treatment, is, unfortunately, a very difficult one for both patient and family. You may find some answers to the psychological problems that such stresses inevitably throw up on pp.130-148.

How long will I have to wait for treatment?

Patients with cancer invariably get priority preference to hospital beds so the time between diagnosis and hospital admission should only be a matter of days.

Like any organization, the medical profession has its fair share of faults and I think that probably one of its greatest failings is often not appreciating the stresses and strains put upon the patient who is entering hospital, perhaps for the first time. Not only is the knowledge to the patient that he has cancer a very great worry but this anxiety is increased by the fact that he is entering the unknown world of a hospital. The patient's fear of these two unknowns can be immense and this is sometimes not fully appreciated by the medical staff. After all, the hospital is their normal working environment, and it is sometimes difficult, especially for the more inexperienced members among them, to appreciate that walking into a hospital can be a very stressful experience for a patient who may be entering a ward for the first time. I am glad to say, however, that attitudes are changing and in recent years a much greater appreciation of patients' needs has been recognized.

What will happen when I get to the hospital?

If you are called into hospital by letter, you may find an accompanying booklet telling you all about the hospital and suggesting what you should bring with you in terms of toiletries or clothes. If you do not receive such a booklet and don't know what to take with you, then the ward will be only too glad to receive a telephone call from you. One of the ward staff will be able to tell you over the phone what to bring and the best time to arrive on your day of admission. Do not be afraid to ask any questions. You will find that, from the start, the staff will be very friendly and only too glad to help.

If at all possible, I feel that it is always best to be accompanied by someone when going into hospital. This is for two reasons: first, it will give you a degree of moral support; second, your friend or relative can fetch any things that you find you have forgotten and bring them to you later on in the day. If you think that you are going to have difficulties getting to the hospital, contact your GP, who may be able to arrange for an ambulance or a hospital car to get you there.

When you walk on to the ward, you will be greeted by one of several people. You may be met by the ward sister. She is the senior nurse on the ward, with day-to-day control over all aspects of ward management and the nurses who work on the ward, and also works closely with your consultant and the rest of the medical team. On the other hand, you may be greeted by the ward sister's deputy, a staff nurse, or by a state-enrolled nurse – another form of trained nurse who will also have had much experience in ward work. Alternatively, you may come across a student nurse. This is a nurse who is still in training but who nevertheless will be under the close supervision of either the ward sister or one of her staff nurses.

Sometimes you will not be met by a nurse at all but, rather, by someone known as the ward clerk. It is her responsibility to see to various aspects of administration such as preparing the patient's notes for admission, giving out and collecting patient menus and generally being on hand to sort out and look after the patient's notes and X-rays.

It is possible that, if you have been up to the ward before – say, for your initial tests – you may have met one or all of these people already. If not, rest assured – they are all very much caring professionals. If you have any worries or doubts concerning your admission or treatment, feel free to ask any of them any questions you like.

The worst thing that you can do on a hospital ward is to bottle up your fears and worries. By talking them through with someone else, you will normally find that they will seem much less of a burden.

You will then be shown to your bed on the ward. The relative or friend who has come with you will be able to sit with you for a few minutes but will then be asked to leave and the formal process of admission will begin.

What does the admission process involve?

The first person to come to see you will be a nurse. Recently, a procedure known as the 'nursing process' has been introduced into hospitals. This involves assigning one nurse to a particular patient or group of patients. The idea behind this is to try to achieve a continuity in nursing care so that from the moment of admission you will be looked after, where possible, by the same nurse.

This system has many advantages and has much to commend it. Often, it is only very subtle changes in a patient's overall condition that can indicate that a medical problem is occurring. Such changes can readily be appreciated by someone who has cared for the patient right from the start.

Having introduced herself and having asked if there are any pressing questions that you want answered, your nurse will then go about the process of admission. This will entail attaching to your wrist a plastic tag on which your name, your ward and your hospital number will be written. This tag is a very important means of identification and if you ever find that it has slipped off your wrist you must inform the nursing staff immediately. The nurse will then take a detailed nursing history, which may include medical details but will concentrate on your daily living activities and your life at home. In doing this, she will be trying to identify whether you have any problems which she may be able to help you solve while you are in hospital. She may be able to tell you what day your operation is likely to be and what is likely to happen beforehand: for example, when your consultant will be doing his ward round before the operation and any necessary pre-operative preparations that you will require. At some stage, later on the same day, you will be visited by the houseman – the junior doctor on your medical team. He will take from you a detailed medical history and will examine you, even though this may well have been done when you were originally admitted for your initial tests. He will enlarge upon the type of operation or treatment that you will be having though he may leave the exact details of this to your consultant. Finally, he will ask you to sign your consent form for the operation.

Don't forget, if you have any questions, always put them to the doctors and nurses at any stage. They will be only too glad to give you any answers that will make your stay in hospital less stressful.

Your next contact with your medical team will be your consultant's ward round. During this, your consultant may well be accompanied by an entourage which may, at first sight, seem intimidating. But amongst these people will be vital members of the backup team.

For instance, the physiotherapist, who will be responsible for an important part of your post-operative recovery, a medical social worker who you will be able to speak to after your operation and who will be able to sort out any social or convalescence problems you may have. As well as these members of the medical team there might well be junior doctors and medical students.

Try, under these circumstances, to concentrate on your consultant and what he is saying to you. The main function of his ward round is to make sure that all the other members of his team have done their job. By the time that he has reached you he will be in a position to tell you precisely what he proposes to do. He will probably re-examine that particular part of anatomy that is affected by the cancer and then explain to you what sort of operation or treatment he proposes for you.

At this stage many patients feel very intimidated and find themselves unable to ask questions. This is an entirely understandable reaction. If you do feel constrained to ask questions, once the ward round has finished you can always ask the ward sister or a doctor on your consultant's medical team to enlarge upon the points that he made.

Remember, nobody minds you asking questions. Indeed, all members of the medical team will welcome them.

The ward clerk will then come round with the menus and show you how to fill them in. I am glad to say that hospital food has undergone a revolutionary change and, unless your condition specifically excludes it, you will normally have a fairly wide choice.

Will I have a problem sleeping in hospital?

Your first night in hospital may be a problem. In fact, sleeping in hospitals generally can be a problem. Not only are you in a strange bed, in strange surroundings and naturally concerned about your forthcoming treatment but you may also be disturbed by the inevitable background noises of the ward.

If you think that you may have trouble getting to sleep you can ask the houseman to write you up for a sleeping tablet so that it is available should you need it. Your doctor may do this for you, routinely. Such sleeping tablets, for a short period of time, are not addictive and you will not have to continue them when you leave the hospital and go home.

Is there anything else I should know about hospital routine?

Smoking will not be allowed on the ward but if you simply cannot get through a day without smoking you will be shown areas, off the ward, where you can have a quick smoke if you wish.

As far as radios and televisions are concerned, these will always be provided on a communal basis on the ward. Nowadays, many people bring their own radios and televisions into hospital although they are encouraged to use headphones or earplugs in order not to disturb other patients. All wards will have a ward telephone and ready access to daily papers, magazines and library books.

What will be involved in the preparations for my operation?

Steps will be taken before your operation to ensure that post-operative complications do not arise. One such complication, known as deep vein thrombosis, occurs when blood clots form in the veins of the legs. To prevent this, you will pre-operatively be encouraged to be as mobile as possible and taught simple exercises to perform after surgery. You may also be given special elastic supportive stockings to wear, which will significantly reduce the incidence of post-operative deep vein thrombosis.

If you have chest problems or difficulty in breathing, the physio-therapist will come and see you before your operation to give you breathing exercises.

You will also be visited by your anaesthetist – the person who will 'put you to sleep'. His main concern will be the state of your heart and lungs. It is important that he examines you carefully before the operation so that he can spot any potential problems that might arise while you are under the anaesthetic. He may suggest that an electrical examination (known as an ECG or electrocardiogram) be done. This does not mean to say that he has found anything wrong with your heart, it is simply routine before any major operation. If you have not had a chest X-ray up till now, he will probably request that this also be done.

Then, having assessed you from the point of view of the anaesthetic he will write up a particular premedication for you, which will be given just before your operation. By this stage you will almost certainly know on what day your operation is going to be and whether the operation is going to be in the morning or in the afternoon.

What will happen on the day of operation?

On the day of your operation you will be what is known as 'nil by mouth'. This means that you are not allowed to eat or drink anything.

If, for any reason, you are offered something to eat or drink, politely refuse and ask the ward sister, her staff nurse or the houseman whether or not you have done the right thing.

About an hour and a half before your operation you may be asked to bathe, to go to the lavatory and put on an operation gown. Then, an hour before your operation you will be given your pre-medication. This is normally given in the form of an intramuscular injection, either in your arm or your buttock and will have the effect of drying up the secretions in your mouth and throat, which will make it technically much easier and safer for the anaesthetist to administer the anaesthetic. It will also leave you with a feeling of general well-being and will tend to eliminate any worries that you may have had up till then.

After this, you will be taken down to theatre, where you will probably see some familiar faces though they will be in unfamiliar clothes and surroundings. Your consultant and his team will be there. The anaesthetist will also be there as will your nurse, who will have come with you from the ward. Once more you will be thoroughly checked. These checks may seem tedious, but they are vital to make sure that the right patient is being operated on in the right operating theatre at the right time. When everything is ready, your anaesthetist will then tell you that he is going to put you to sleep. This is done by placing a small needle in the back of your hand. He will inject a quick-acting anaesthetic and within five to ten seconds you will find yourself going off to sleep.

41

What happens when I come around from the anaesthetic?

Extraordinarily, the first thing that you may probably think is that you are still waiting for your operation. This is a very common phenomenon. What will probably make you gradually aware that you have had an operation will be the realization that you have an intravenous drip going into the back of your hand. This is a very necessary part of your post-operative treatment. For some time after your operation, and especially if you have had an operation on your abdomen, it will be dangerous to take fluids by mouth. Fluid balance and bodily hydration are vital not only for recovery but also for normal physiological functions. The drip will consequently be kept going until such time as it is safe for you to take fluids by mouth.

Do not worry if, when you look up, you see that you are receiving a blood transfusion. After cancer operations, this is often quite normal because during the operation there is often a certain amount of blood loss and, rather than allow your body to make up the blood loss naturally, it is often best to give you a blood transfusion because the less anaemic you are the more efficient will be the healing processes of your body. It may be worth noting here that, with the increasing concern about AIDS, all blood is carefully screened before it is used for transfusions.

For the first 24 hours after your operation, and especially if you are receiving a transfusion, you will find that the nurses will regularly come round to check your pulse, temperature and blood pressure. This is a normal procedure for post-operative patients.

As you gradually come around from your anaesthetic you may begin to experience a certain amount of pain from the operation site. If you do, tell the nurses at once and they will be able to give you an intramuscular injection of a pain killing drug. Do not suffer pain in silence. There will always be a certain amount of post-operative discomfort, but no patient should be allowed to suffer pain post-operatively.

What will happen after the immediate post-operative period?

How your post-operative progress will unfold will depend upon your own individual situation. In general terms it is now medical policy to get patients mobilized as soon as possible since this decreases the risk of deep vein thrombosis and respiratory complications. You may even, on the first day after your operation, be allowed to sit out of bed even though you still have an intravenous drip. As well as being encouraged to move as much as possible, you will receive a visit from your physiotherapist. She will give you a series of simple exercises designed to ensure that the muscles of your body maintain their tone and strength. These muscles can easily lose their strength if they are inactive and if this happens it can sometimes take many weeks for them to regain their former condition. The physiotherapist will also give you some breathing exercises to enable you to fully expand your chest. If necessary she will percuss your chest to loosen any secretions that are making breathing difficult. Remember, throughout your post-operative period, if you are experiencing any discomfort, let the medical staff know immediately.

According to your consultant's instructions, you will have the dressings on your wound changed during the post-operative period. Sometimes, when the dressing comes off for the first time and you see the incisional scar, the sight of it can be a great worry to you. It is important to bear in mind, therefore, that at this stage in the immediate post-operative period, the incisions and their stitches always look very much at their worst. The end result will normally be a scar that is barely visible.

You may also find bits of polythene or rubber tubing coming out of the wound. These are known as wound drains, and allow for any fluid that has collected under the skin and under the incision to drain away. They will be removed during the post-operative period – a painless procedure.

After a variable amount of time you will find that your drip will be removed and that your mobility will gradually improve and you will be allowed to do more for yourself. You will be visited on a regular daily basis by the houseman, and will also be seen by your consultant on his routine ward rounds.

Once you are over the immediate post-operative period your consultant will tell you about your operation, though he will probably still be unable precisely to predict the long-term outlook until you see him in the outpatients department two or three weeks after your discharge. By this time he will have the pathology results of the tissue that he removed from you during the operation.

The time that you spend in hospital is a time for operative recovery. It is a time for you to let your doctors do the worrying. Your main priority should be to concentrate on getting better.

How should I approach convalescence?

As you begin to feel better it is important for you to look to the future, your convalescent period. Ask your consultant on his ward round when he expects to discharge you from the ward. Once you have a rough date, you can then start to make arrangements.

The choice will normally fall between going straight home or going to a convalescent home for a period of recuperation. If you think you are going to have problems making arrangements, you can discuss these problems with the ward sister and the medical social worker. They will take down details of your medical condition and your social circumstances and will normally be able to arrange a suitable plan for your convalescence if you so wish.

Eventually, the day will come for your discharge. When it does, have three things absolutely clear in your mind. First, be sure of where and for how long you are going to convalesce, and the date for your first appointment to see your consultant in the outpatients clinic. Second, if you are on a course of tablets make sure that the hospital gives you a supply of these tablets to tide you over at home or during your convalescence. Thirdly, if you have not been given specific instructions as to what you should or should not be doing, ask either the ward sister or the doctors for specific 'dos and don'ts'. Following abdominal operations and gynaecological procedures, for instance, lifting heavy weights is definitely forbidden.

What will happen when I go back to the outpatients department?

By the time that you go back to the outpatients department you will almost certainly be feeling very much better and well on the road to recovery. You will again see your consultant, who will examine you and make sure that the wound site is healing properly even though it will already have been examined during your period of convalescence by a district nurse, whose visits will have been arranged either by your GP or by the medical social worker.

When he has finished his examination your consultant will then tell you what was found at the operation, what was done, and how he intends to proceed in the future.

By this time he will have an idea of the long-term outlook for your case and I think that it is important at this stage for you to ask him, in specific terms, what these are. You quite naturally do not want to hear bad news but it is important for you to know what the future holds so that you can plan for all eventualities. Though whether or not you wish to discuss these questions is entirely up to you.

Your consultant will also probably explain to you that although your surgical treatment has been successfully concluded you need further treatment to eliminate any cancer that may have spread before it was possible to do the operation.

In essence these further forms of treatment can either be radiotherapy or chemotherapy, though in some cases these treatments are used alone, in place of surgery.

What does radiotherapy entail?

When we discussed the basic features of cancerous tissue, I stated that it was the uncontrolled and haphazard division of cells that produced an area of cancerous tissue within normal tissue. As these cells reproduce in a haphazard and uncontrolled way, the cancerous growth gradually enlarges with subsequent local and general effects on the body. The aim of radiotherapy treatment is to damage the reduplicating control mechanisms within the cancer cells themselves. This is achieved by means of high-energy radiation, which can be focused with great precision upon an area of cancer tissue.

These high-energy rays are quite invisible and receiving them is an entirely painless procedure. As well as inhibiting the division of cancer cells, under certain circumstances, radiotherapy will actually cause shrinkage of the cancer tissue. As I have mentioned, it is often the expanding cancer tissue that can cause the pain that is sometimes associated with cancer. The ability of these high-energy radiations to shrink the offending cancer can give pain relief.

So radiotherapy is used, on the one hand, to kill cancerous cells and on the other to shrink cancerous tissues. This relieves such symptoms as pain or obstruction of internal organs.

Radiotherapy can be given in two ways: externally or internally. In external radiotherapy, the radiation being beamed from, in some cases, a large machine that can initially appear rather intimidating. With internal radiotherapy, on the other hand, the radioactive source may actually be implanted or inserted into the cancerous area.

Radiotherapy may be given either before or after your operation, the time being different for certain cancers. If given post-operatively, you will go to the radiotherapy department as soon as you have recovered from the operation. There you will meet the consultant radiotherapist, the doctor who will be in charge of your treatment. At this first visit he will go over the details of your case and will explain the part that radiotherapy will have to play in your continuing treatment. This may be to prevent the tumour growing any larger, so reducing any pain or discomfort it may be giving you, or it may be to eradicate cancer within certain lymph nodes that has arisen as a result of spread from the primary cancer.

The reason for irradiating lymph nodes may seem, at first sight, to be rather strange. When talking about the basic forms of cancer and the spread of cancer, I mentioned that lymph nodes were an integral part of the immune system and were a part of the body's defence mechanism in fighting cells that looked as though they were about to become cancerous. This is certainly the case. But in certain circumstances, not only can the lymph nodes become overwhelmed by cancerous cells but they can become staging posts for these cells, helping their eventual spread. This is one way in which secondary cancers, or metastases, can occur. Once the lymph nodes become overwhelmed by these cancerous cells their function becomes compromised, and under such circumstances it is best to irradiate such lymph nodes, to prevent the spread of the cancer.

Your consultant radiotherapist will decide what sort of radiotherapy you are to receive from all the data that he has available. This will include your pre-operative investigations together with the operative findings and the reports from the pathological specimens that were taken at operation. He will then examine you, paying particular attention to the area of your body that is to receive treatment. The reason for this is that in almost all cases in order to be focused on the tissue that is to be treated the radiation will have to pass through the overlying skin. This area of skin can often be slightly affected by the therapy, though radiotherapy does not cause burns. This will normally simply take the form of reddening but it is still important for the radiotherapist to make sure that this area of skin is in the best possible condition before beginning the treatment. He will, therefore, try to avoid areas of skin which may have been involved in the operation site. He will ask you to be particularly careful to avoid the area of skin through which the radiotherapy will be given when you are washing though, in certain circumstances, this may be difficult.

The area of skin that is to be treated will normally be outlined with a coloured dye, which allows the radiotherapist to site his instruments accurately and will also act as a reminder for you when washing. The dye tends not to rub off and should never be washed off until the course of treatment is over.

Once your consultant radiotherapist has fully assessed the situation he will be in a position to tell you what form of radiotherapy you will be receiving, how many sessions you will need and over what period of time you will be receiving them. Treatments are normally given on a daily basis and they may last from anything between one and four weeks depending on your requirements. The reason for this somewhat extended period is that it is generally considered best to give frequent, small doses of radiation rather than large doses over a shorter period of time. Frequent, small doses will ensure that the cancerous tissues receive the maximum dose of radiation while the overlying skin and the normal healthy tissue surrounding the cancer will be relatively unaffected.

When you return to the radiotherapy department for your first session of treatment you will find that the person in control of the radiotherapy apparatus will be a technician working under the supervision of your consultant radiotherapist.

You will be asked to get undressed and will be taken into a large room containing the radiotherapy apparatus. At first sight this may appear daunting but do not be worried by its size and scale. Radiotherapy is a completely painless treatment. The size of the machinery is mainly due to the fact that you and it have to be positioned in accurate apposition. For this to occur you both have to move around each other and it is the mechanics of this operation that involves the bulk of the machinery.

As to receiving the treatment, this is simplicity itself. You will be positioned precisely and areas of your body surrounding the site to be radiated will be protected with lead shields. The treatment itself is given over a relatively short period of time, a matter of minutes. When it is over you will be able to get dressed and return home.

Patients are often worried that they may in some way be a danger to their friends and family when they have received radiation. This is not the case. You are definitely not radioactive when you have received external radiation therapy and are in no way a danger to anybody about you.

The number of visits you make to the radiotherapy department will depend upon the dose of radiation that you require. During your visits you will probably see your consultant radiotherapist and he will almost certainly give you a final examination when your course of radiotherapy is completed. You may well see him on a fairly long-term basis because if there are any recurrences of cancer, for instance, in the bones, it will probably mean that you will need a further course of radiotherapy.

What are the side-effects of radiotherapy?

Sometimes it is difficult to distinguish the side-effects of radiotherapy from the effects of your operation and chemotherapy which you may be receiving at the same time as your radiotherapy. However, it is not at all uncommon to feel tired following radiotherapy. Together with this tiredness there is also sometimes a general loss of appetite, and a change in bowel function – in particular you may find that diarrhoea is a troublesome problem. This can be easily treated by changing your diet or taking anti-diarrhoeal treatment prescribed by your doctor.

Radiotherapy may also affect the upper part of your digestive tract, especially if the treatment has been given either to your chest or to regions of your neck. This may leave you with difficulty in eating or swallowing. Tell your GP and your radiotherapist about these problems. A change in diet to one of rather more liquid content will usually improve the situation.

Radiotherapy is normally given on an outpatient basis but, either for convenience of travel or for closer monitoring, you may be asked to remain as an in-patient. Again, do not worry if this happens. This does not denote a particular seriousness of your condition. It just means that for various reasons the radiotherapy treatment will be best received in hospital.

If you do have any side-effects from radiotherapy these will normally clear up within a month following the completion of your course of treatment. If they do not, go and see your GP.

What is chemotherapy?

Chemotherapy is the use of drugs to either damage or kill cancer cells. Like the other forms of cancer treatment, chemotherapy has advantages and disadvantages. Its main advantage is that drugs can reach all parts of the body, including areas that may be inaccessible to radiotherapy or surgery. The major disadvantages of chemotherapy are that these necessarily toxic drugs tend, in the main, to be non-specific in their effects and can damage normal cells as well as cancerous cells. The drugs are extremely effective in eliminating cells that divide rapidly, which is one of the characteristics of cancerous cells. But there are also other non-cancerous cells in the body which divide quite rapidly, in particular the cells of the bone marrow (which manufacture the constituents of the blood, red blood cells, white blood cells and platelets). So these chemo-therapeutic agents must be used with caution to avoid serious side-effects on these healthy areas.

It is because of the particular problems associated with chemotherapy that the speciality of medical oncology has arisen. Medical oncologists are doctors who specialize in the medical treatment of cancer and they will explain the side-effects of these chemotherapeutic agents to you. In effect, this is a careful balance between, on the one hand, using these chemotherapeutic agents to eliminate cancerous tissue and, on the other, minimizing the side-effects that these agents can sometimes have. You and your medical oncologist will decide what is acceptable to you.

Most people prefer to accept these side-effects in the knowledge that, in the long run, their cancer, if not entirely eliminated, will at least be held at bay. I shall go into specific details about the particular types of chemotherapy that are used for individual cancers in the next section of the book.

What are the side-effects of chemotherapy?

As mentioned earlier, chemotherapeutic agents can cause suppression of the bone marrow. This can cause a lowering of the red blood cells, white blood cells and platelets. A lowering of red blood cells means that you may become anaemic – a condition which can give symptoms of fatigue, breathlessness and occasional dizzy spells.

Anaemia can also be a symptom of cancer, however. The combination of cancer, anaemia and chemotherapeutic anaemia can be quite substantial and may mean your having to go into hospital for a blood transfusion.

Platelets are responsible for blood clotting and a deficiency will allow a tendency to bruising or bleeding. If you find that you are bruising easily or that, when you cut yourself, you tend to bleed for rather longer than usual, tell your doctor immediately.

White cells are part of the immune system, which is responsible for combating infection. A lowering of the white cell count will mean that you are more vulnerable to infection. Any infection that you contract while you are receiving chemotherapy, therefore, should immediately be reported. In some cases the infection will have to be treated with a course of antibiotics.

As I mentioned earlier, chemotherapeutic agents tend to selectively attack rapidly dividing cells. One group of such cells are the cells of the hair follicles. This can mean that chemotherapy sometimes results in the loss of hair, though scalp hair can be temporarily substituted with a wig. In almost all cases the lost hair will regrow although the texture of the new hair may be slightly different.

Another group of cells that are always rapidly dividing are the cells that line the digestive tract. Such lining cells can be affected by chemotherapy, resulting in diarrhoea, though your doctor will be able to give you medication that will give symptomatic improvement for this problem.

At the upper end of your digestive tract the linings of your mouth and gullet known as the mucous membranes can become sore or ulcerated. Sometimes little white patches can form on these mucous membranes. This is a fungal infection commonly known as thrush. If you have this problem an antifungal agent called nystatin will eliminate the fungus.

Chemotherapeutic agents may also upset the lining of both your stomach and your duodenum, resulting in loss of appetite, nausea and actual vomiting. Vomiting can be a serious problem and should not be under-estimated, especially in children receiving chemotherapy where a major problem can be dehydration.

If you are undergoing chemotherapy you may also find that you are beginning to experience tingling sensations in your skin, particularly in your fingers and your toes. The technical term for this is paraesthesia. It may be due either to an allergic response to a particular drug or to a direct effect of the chemotherapy on the nerves that travel near the surface of the skin in the extremities. This is known as a peripheral neuropathy.

Superimposed upon these problems you may discover that your arms and your legs appear to be becoming weaker, known as myopathy.

Once your chemotherapy treatment has finished, however, these side-effects will normally disappear.

One area where chemotherapy has to be used with great caution is in relation to the reproductive organs. There may be no outward manifestations of immediate side-effects of chemotherapy in these areas but long-term problems can arise. In the case of pregnant women, for example, the developing foetus can be damaged and may show abnormalities at birth. Under these circumstances the use of chemotherapy in pregnancy is necessarily a very specialized subject and in the rare cases where it is required will be very carefully monitored.

As for the effects upon the ovaries and the testicles, chemotherapy can sometimes result in sterility and this problem must be weighed against the benefits of the treatment.

What form does chemotherapy take?

This treatment is given in the form of a tablet or intravenous infusion. If you are receiving your chemotherapy orally, this can usually be done on an outpatient basis though it will require your attending the hospital outpatients clinic for the course of treatment to be monitored. Your consultant will be looking for evidence that the chemotherapy is working and also checking that adverse side-effects do not arise, and if they do arise, are treated swiftly.

By its very nature intravenous chemotherapy normally has to be given while you are in hospital. Sometimes it will necessitate an overnight stay because, following your infusion, you may feel nauseous or unwell and it is advisable for you to be somewhere where these problems can be treated.

Features and treatment of specific cancers

What is breast cancer?

This is an important question because it goes a long way to an understanding not only of what breast cancer entails but also of the problems associated with the diagnosis and treatment of this disease.

Breast cancer is a blanket term referring to many sorts of specific cancers that can arise in breast tissue. Some of these cancers are more serious than others. The best way to understand the basic nature of breast cancer is to consider the structure of the breast and then to discuss how the various tissues within it function.

The most important structures, from a functional point of view, are the breast lobules. There are many thousands of these lobules scattered throughout the breast. Each lobule is made up of a little nest of cells, the function of which is to produce milk. The milk that is produced in the lobules flows into a fine network of small tubes known as lactiferous ductules, which, as they pass through the substance of the breast tissue, converge upon the nipple. Surrounding these ductules are specialized muscle cells called myoepithelial cells. When these myoepithelial cells are stimulated, their contraction causes the milk which has been collected in the ductules to become available to a suckling baby at the nipple. So, the structure of breast tissue is designed for its function: milk production.

Breast tissue is covered by skin and overlies the muscles of the chest wall and, in between the lobules, the main bulk of the breast is made up of fatty tissue. These tissues are constantly changing – first at puberty and then again during pregnancy and after the menopause. These changes take place not only over a lifetime but also during each 28-day menstrual cycle, and they are directly influenced by hormones.

Hormones are chemicals produced by the endocrine glands. The main endocrine glands concerned with breast development and growth are the pituitary gland in the brain and specialized endocrine cells in the ovary.

Other endocrine glands lend support, these being the thyroid gland and the adrenal gland. At various specific times these glands secrete their hormones into the bloodstream, bringing about the changes in the breast at puberty, during pregnancy and the menopause as well as the changes during the 28-day menstrual cycle.

Let's take these individually and see how the hormones act on the breast tissue in each case.

Firstly, the developing adolescent breast. At puberty, the specialized endocrine cells in the ovary produce a hormone called oestrogen. This is carried by the bloodstream to the breast tissue, causing enlargement of the lobules and ductules, which results in the fully formed mature, female breast. This is an example of what is known as the development of a secondary sexual characteristic.

During pregnancy a further endocrine gland is formed, the placenta. Specialized endocrine cells are formed within the placenta. These cells secrete large amounts of the hormones oestrogen and progesterone into the bloodstream which, when taken up by the breast tissue, are responsible for the formation of milk in the breast lobules. This is the reason for the characteristic breast enlargement in pregnancy. When the newborn babe sucks the mother's nipple this stimulation causes the pituitary gland to release a hormone known as oxytocin which in turn stimulates the myoepithelial cells surrounding the ductules that are filled with milk. In this elegant manner milk is expelled from the breast, at the nipple, to satisfy the suckling baby.

At the menopause, the endocrine cells in the ovary begin to disappear and, as a consequence, the oestrogen secretion falls away. This causes the lobules and ductules to be replaced by fatty tissue.

So, throughout a woman's lifetime, the changing structure and function of the breast tissue is very much under the direct control of hormones. This is particularly the case during each menstrual cycle, when a hormone from the pituitary gland called prolactin and two hormones from the ovary, progesterone and oestrogen, stimulate growth followed by tissue regression of the ductules and lobules. This monthly cyclical change demonstrates the ever-changing nature of the tissues within the breast. And it is because of these cyclical changes that problems can often arise in deciding whether or not a particular lump is benign or malignant.

Now that we have gone over the basic groundwork in understanding what structures are found within the breast and how these structures grow and develop under the direct influence of hormones we are in a better position to understand the basic nature of breast cancer.

Cancer of the breast normally manifests itself as a lump, but one thing that I cannot emphasize too strongly is that all breast lumps are not cancerous. The majority of breast lumps are non-cancerous. That is not to say that each and every breast lump should not be taken seriously. Of course it should, and if you notice a breast lump you should report it to your doctor immediately. But the good news is that the likelihood of that breast lump being benign is far greater than of being malignant.

What types of breast lumps are there?

One of the commonest is known as a fibroadenoma. Fibroadenomas are probably the commonest form of breast lump and are entirely harmless. They arise from the lining cells of the lobules. Although the cells that produce these fibroadenomas do so by reduplicating themselves in an uncontrolled way, their mode of growth is not cancerous.

Another very common form of benign breast lump is known as fibroadenosis, which used to be called chronic mastitis. This condition is characterized by diffuse painful lumpy areas within the breast tissue. It is caused by proliferation of the lobule cells, probably due to an imbalance of the hormones oestrogen and progesterone. Like the fibroadenoma, fibroadenosis is non-cancerous.

Like any tissue, the breast is susceptible to infection, and the general term for this infection in the breast is mastitis. While breast feeding, infection can be introduced into the breast tissue by way of the nipple. This sets up an infection within the lobules which is experienced as a tense painful swelling within the breast tissue. Such swellings have nothing to do with cancer.

The three benign breast conditions which I have mentioned, fibroadenoma, fibroadenosis and mastitis, tend to occur in the younger age groups. But there is one other important benign tumour which should be mentioned, which tends to occur in women of 30 and above. This is known as a solitary breast cyst. It is often extremely difficult to differentiate these solitary cysts from breast cancer.

There are also rarer, benign breast conditions but I have just mentioned four of the commonest types, to demonstrate two basic facts. Namely, that not all breast lumps or tumours are malignant but that, by the same token, they should not automatically be assumed to be benign.

Now to pass on to malignant tumours, or carcinomas, of the breast. The vast majority of these cancers arise from the cells that line the lobules and the ductules. Why these cells are particularly liable to cancerous changes is not known. Neither is it known why some breast cancers can be cured whilst others may become progressive.

There is, however, a method of ascertaining which cancers are more likely to be more progressive than others. This is by dividing those cancers that develop in the lobules and ductules into those which remain contained within them and those which tend to spread beyond their borders. Cancers that remain within the ductules and the lobules are known as non-invasive cancers; cancers that extend beyond these areas are described as being invasive. This distinction is important because the long-term outcome of cancer treatment can, to a certain extent, be predicted from knowing whether or not the cancer is invasive or non-invasive.

Within the breast tissue are lymphatic channels which drain into the lymph nodes found in clusters around the breast tissue, in particular in the armpit region known as the axilla. If cancer cells are found in these lymph nodes then definite spread is known to have taken place. What I have just described, in simple terms, is known as staging.

The staging of cancers is important both for determining the probable outcome as well as deciding what forms of further treatment will be needed in terms of radiotherapy and chemotherapy.

Staging is assessed by looking at the tumour tissue both with the naked eye and also under the microscope. If the tumour is contained within the lobules and ductules and its cells do not appear to be growing particularly quickly then such a cancer is said to be at an early stage of development.

The next stage is where the cancer cells are seen to involve parts of the breast tissue outside the ductules and the lobules.

A more serious stage is reached when the cancer cells have reached the local lymph nodes.

The last stage is the most serious. This is where the cancer cells reach other parts of the body such as the bones and the liver. Such sites of cancer spread are referred to as being metastatic.

What causes breast cancer?

There are various types of breast cancer, some rarer than others. It follows that since there are many different types of breast cancer there is necessarily no simple, single causative agent. The cause of breast cancer is a multifactorial problem. In other words, a series of influences both from within the body and without (i.e. the environmental influences) combine to produce the circumstances under which this cancer can develop.

What are the factors that make it more likely for cancer to develop within the breast?

Let us first consider the evidence as to whether or not cancer of the breast is an inherited phenomenon. There is a widely held view that inheritance or genetic predisposition is a risk factor in the development of breast cancer. In other words, if a close relative such as a mother or a sister develops breast cancer, the chances of another sister developing breast cancer are slightly more than if she were a member of the general population. If a female relative develops breast cancer before her menopause then the chances of other female relatives acquiring the disease are also slightly increased. But I must emphasize that in these two groups of women the chances of acquiring breast cancer are statistically only marginally increased over those of the general population. There is, however, a very rare group of women who are particularly prone to developing breast cancer. These are daughters of mothers who developed cancer in both breasts before the age of 35.

So, there is some evidence of an inherited risk factor. However, environmental influences must always be taken into consideration when assessing inheritance risk factors. This is because mothers tend to bring up their daughters in much the same environment in which they themselves have lived. Their dietary habits are similar. Their social habits are likely to be the same, including the age at which they first become pregnant, the number of children they have, whether or not they use contraception and whether they have had hormone replacement therapy for the menopause. Also, the locality in which they live may be higher in background radiation. These are just a few examples to show how difficult it is to unravel direct genetic evidence of a supposed genetic predisposition in the development of any cancer.

Taking these inheritance risk factors just one step further, the subject can be expanded into one of geographic location together with certain racial customs. Studies of such factors are known as epidemiological surveys.

Let us now look at certain populations and in particular at the instance of breast cancers in these populations. Figures show that breast cancer is a more common problem in Western women living in European countries and in North America. In Japan, however, the disease is rare. But, once again, looking at these figures more closely, the epidemiological evidence gives a rather more complicated picture because two distinct groups of Japanese women can be identified. The first are Japanese women living in Japan; the second group are the Japanese women and their daughters who emigrated to the USA. In this second group of Japanese women, breast cancer is much more common than in those Japanese women living in

Japan. The rates of breast cancer occurring in second generation Japanese women in the USA closely approximates those of breast cancer in the general female American population.

So the question has often been asked: is there something about the Western lifestyle that predisposes to breast cancer? But the answer to this tantalizing question is as yet unknown.

Does diet have an effect on breast cancer?

Studies have been made of the relative dietary constituents of affluent Western societies, where breast cancer is more prominent, and the dietary habits of countries where breast cancer is less common. It has emerged that in affluent societies the consumption of saturated fats, so-called animal fats, is higher than in the less affluent societies where the predominant dietary fats are vegetable or unsaturated fats. Studies in animals have also shown that animals fed on saturated fats are more likely to develop breast cancer than those fed on unsaturated fats. In this respect, it is interesting to note that obesity after the menopause has been associated with an increased incidence of breast cancer.

In affluent societies the intake of protein is much higher than in non-affluent societies. For this reason some surveys have implicated a high-protein diet as being a risk factor in developing breast cancer.

I think it is fair to say, however, that at the present time there is no completely positive evidence that fats or proteins, in varying quantities, contribute to the direct causation of breast cancer.

Having said that, one important point to emerge from these dietary studies is that in the future dietary factors may well be shown to be one part of the multifactorial cause of cancer.

Can hormones contribute to breast cancer?

You will recall that I explained how the anatomical structure of the breast can be greatly modified by hormones, particularly hormones produced by the pituitary gland and the ovary. I have also mentioned how these hormones can cause considerable changes in cells with potential for reduplication, namely the lining cells of the ductules and the lobules. It is reasonable, therefore, to look at various stages in the life cycle of the female breast, to see if any of these hormonal influences has a direct bearing on the development of cancer.

Let us first of all look at menstruation. There is evidence to indicate that the earlier menstruation begins, the greater the risk of developing breast cancer later in life. But there are many other factors that must be taken into account. Menstruation tends to start much earlier in affluent Western societies than in non-Western societies, where many factors contribute to the onset of what, in Western society, would be considered to be delayed puberty.

Is there a relationship between breast feeding, pregnancy and breast cancer?

In women over 30 who are childless, there is an increased risk of breast cancer, whereas women who have had one or more pregnancies in their twenties are less likely, in later life, to develop the disease.

Looking more closely at this group of child-bearing women a further division can be made between women who breast-feed their babies and those women who bottle-feed their babies.

For many years it has been claimed that breast-feeding protects against breast cancer. Why this should be so is not clear, though it would appear that there is an element of truth in this assumption. It is increasingly believed that it is not so much breast-feeding that confers what might loosely be called protection against breast cancer but, rather, pregnancy itself. A certain amount of breast cancer protection appears to come from carrying the pregnancy to full term. There is evidence that conception followed by a miscarriage may very slightly increase the risk of breast cancer.

Can other hormonal effects contribute to the development of breast cancer?

The menopause is a time in a woman's life when hormone levels are undergoing fundamental change. When looked at statistically there does not appear to be any evidence to suggest that the menopause necessarily either heralds the advent of cancer or protects against it. It would appear that if cancer is going to develop in the breast then the blueprint for this development has probably been laid down by a series of factors over many years.

There is, however, the problem of artificial hormones – most notably, the contraceptive pill, for inhibiting pregancy, and hormone replacement therapy, for lessening the symptoms and the effects of the menopause. Recently, there have been a series of reports that have pointed to the possibility of the contraceptive pill being a risk factor in breast cancer. As things stand at present, however, there is no concrete evidence to substantiate these claims.

Likewise, there is no evidence that hormone replacement therapy can cause breast cancer in menopausal women. However, recent reports from the USA have suggested that there might be a slightly increased incidence of breast cancer in women receiving hormone replacement therapy over a long period of time (from eight to ten years) though such claims have not as yet been substantiated.

Can viruses cause breast cancer?

When causes of any cancer are being discussed, the possibility that the cancer might be produced by a virus is always mooted. This has certainly been the case for some years where breast cancer is concerned. In certain groups of women who are particularly prone to breast cancer, viral particles have been found by the electron microscope. Similar particles, known as the Bitner Factor, have been shown to cause breast cancer in certain animals. But apart from this rather obscure piece of evidence for a viral cause there are no other concrete facts to suggest that breast cancer is caused by a virus.

Are there any environmental chemicals that can cause breast cancer?

We are all increasingly exposed to a vast number of man-made chemicals both in the atmosphere and in our diets. Many such chemicals are believed to be carcinogenic, or cancer-producing, and it has been suggested that one of these carcinogens may be the cause of breast cancer. Suspicion has been particularly centred on nitrates (used as artificial fertilizers), cyclamates (sweeteners) and other artificial flavourings and food additives. None of these has been specifically shown to cause breast cancer but it is thought that in the future we may discover that certain dietary additives, while not actually causing cancer, may well play an initiating role in the early stages of certain cancers.

What does self-examination of the breast involve?

The following is a précis of the advice given by the Women's National Cancer Control Campaign and is reproduced here with their permission.

Undress to the waist and sit or stand in front of a mirror in a good light. In the first examination you should note the normal size and shape of each breast and the position of the nipples so that you will be aware of any changes that might develop. In subsequent examinations you should look for any inequality in the size or shape of your breasts, or any other change in their appearance.

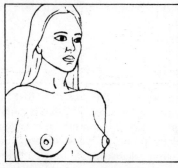

1. LOOK: hands at your sides or on your hips, look carefully at your breasts. Turn from side to side. Look underneath too.

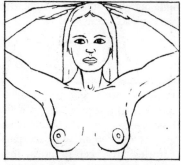

2. LIFT: hands on your head, look for anything unusual, especially around the nipple.

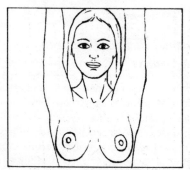

3. STRETCH: arms stretched above your head, look again, particularly around the nipple.

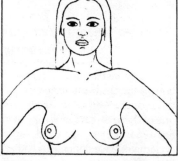

4. PRESS: hands on hips, press inwards until your chest muscles tighten. Look again, especially for any dimpling of the skin.

You have completed the inspection part of the examination and now it is time to feel for any abnormal lumps in the breasts. Again, it is important at the first examination to note the normal consistency of your breasts so that you will be aware of any change in subsequent examinations. Many women who have not yet reached the menopause normally have rather lumpy breasts just before a period and in some this may persist throughout the whole month. This may cause uncertainty at first but with each successive examination it should become easier to decide whether an unusual lump is present. Lie down comfortably on a flat surface, head on a pillow, shoulder slightly raised by a folded towel.

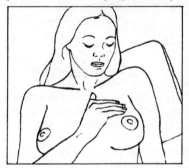

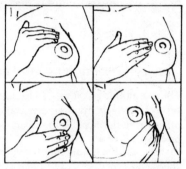

5. Left shoulder raised, feel the left breast with the right hand.

6. Press the breast gently but firmly in towards the body. Work in a spiral, circling out from the nipple. Feel every part.

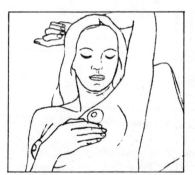

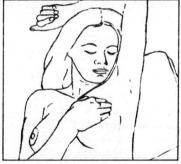

7. Lift arm above your head, elbow bent, repeat the spiral carefully. Feel the outer part of the breast especially.

8. Finish by feeling the tail of the breast towards the armpit. Be thorough. Don't rush.

What are the symptoms of breast cancer?

The following in particular are signs to look out for: any unusual difference in the size or shape of the breasts; a change in the position or appearance of your nipples (does either of them turn in on itself, or point up or outwards unusually? Is there any bleeding or discharge from either nipple?); puckering or dimpling or swelling of the skin surface; an unusual rash on the breast or nipple; unusual prominence of the veins over either breast, any unusual lumps or thickenings of either breast.

Is there anything I can do to prevent breast cancer?

There is nothing you can do to directly prevent the disease. But you can protect yourself by regularly examining your breasts for lumps or any other irregularities. Remember, breast cancer, if detected early, can be cured.

Try to make the examination of your breasts a monthly habit. Immediately following a period would be a suitable time or on the first day of each month if you have had the menopause.

Remember, even if you find a lump or thickening, it will probably be benign. In the unlikely event that it is cancer, your chances will be vastly improved if the diagnosis is made early.

If you have any difficulty following these diagrams, or are unsure about anything, your doctor will be able to help you.

What should I do if I find a lump in my breast?

Let us suppose that, while routinely examining your breast you come across a lump. Or, perhaps – even more importantly – you come across something that you *think* might be a lump.

Under these circumstances you must, without delay, make an appointment to see your doctor. I must emphasize that even if there is some uncertainty in your mind over whether or not you think you have a lump it is important that you go to your GP for his opinion. He will never think that you are wasting his time. So-called 'doubtful' breast lumps are often the reason for breast cancers being diagnosed later rather than sooner.

Don't be worried if, by the time you get to see him, the breast lump appears to have melted away to nothing. With certain varieties of benign breast lump this can and does regularly happen. Your doctor will not feel that you have wasted his time.

It may even be that you don't have anything concrete that you can actually show to your doctor. Your symptoms may, for example, be pain in the breast or, say, discharge from a nipple. Again, I cannot emphasize too strongly that, whatever age you are and however trivial you feel these symptoms are, if you have any sort of a problem or feel that you have noticed a change in either one or both breasts, you *must* seek medical advice.

What will happen when I go and see my doctor with a breast lump?

Under certain circumstances, some more experienced GPs will be able on a mere examination to reassure you that the problem is of a minor nature and requires no further investigation. Most, however, if they find a lump in your breast, will refer you to a consultant surgeon at your local general hospital. They will do this as a safety precaution whether they believe the lump to be malignant or not. Just because you are referred to hospital, therefore, does not mean to say that you have breast cancer. Always remember that most breast lumps are benign, but that in order to exclude the possibility of malignancy, a specialist opinion is necessary.

When you go to the hospital for your outpatients appointment the process of waiting in a crowded area, in unknown territory, together with your silent fears of what the consultant surgeon might have to tell you can be very stressful. But try to remember that although your consultant may be a stranger to you, he will not be a stranger to your GP. Think of the consultant, therefore, as one of your GP's partners. Many of your GP's other patients will have passed this way before.

If, during the initial consultation, you feel either constrained or too nervous to ask questions, you can always go back to your GP to ask him to speak to the consultant on your behalf. He will then be able to answer any questions that were perhaps not broached with your consultant during your visit.

What will happen when I see the consultant?

First, he will take a detailed history of your symptoms and probably ask you a few general questions about you and your health. He will then direct you to the examining room where you will be asked by a nurse to take off your blouse and bra. When you are ready the consultant will begin his examination. He will begin by looking at your breasts to see if they are symmetrical, and to see if there is any nipple retraction or areas of skin retraction over the breast. Then he will ask you to lie down and raise each shoulder in turn while he palpates (feels) each breast. When he finds the breast lump he will examine it more thoroughly. The features that he will be looking for are whether the lump is either fixed to the skin or the underlying tissues. Such characteristics can indicate malignancy. He will also, while he palpates the lump, be trying to assess its size, its shape, and extent as well as its consistency. All these factors will help him to come to a diagnosis. You will also find that he will palpate in and around your armpit. There is a part of the breast tissue known as the axillary tail that extends into this area and also in this region are the lymph nodes that drain lymph from the breast. Apart from the breast itself, both of these areas must also be felt to establish whether or not the cancer has spread there. Having examined your breasts, the consultant may well go on to a general examination to look for other signs of disease. When he has finished his clinical examination, you will be asked to get dressed and come back to the consultant's room. He will then explain, in simple terms, what he has found.

Following this initial examination your consultant may not be in a position to tell you whether or not the lump in your breast is benign or malignant. He will probably explain that, in order to establish a diagnosis beyond doubt, further tests will have to be done. One of these tests may be mammography.

What is mammography?

Mammography is an X-ray investigation of the breasts. The procedure is similiar to having a chest X-ray, but differs in two basic respects: the dosage of X-rays is very low and the procedure takes longer than a normal chest X-ray.

Mammography is completely painless and is done on an outpatient basis in the radiology department. Some doctors feel that mammography should be used for screening rather than for diagnostic purposes. At present, its high costs and the logistical problems that it poses means that it is not readily available for this purpose.

Whether or not you have a mammography, the next stage in the investigation of the breast lump will be taking a biopsy.

What does a breast lump biopsy entail?

This involves taking a small piece of tissue from the lump itself. The tissue can then be examined in the pathology laboratory for any signs of cancerous change. A biopsy sample can be taken in the outpatients department. To obtain it, a small needle is passed through the surface of the skin of the breast and is directed towards the lump. Apart from feeling a small prick as the needle enters the skin, it is a painless procedure.

Instead of this needle biopsy technique, some surgeons are now adopting a different approach, which is to remove part or all of the lump under a general anaesthetic. In the past, it was routine for a patient with a breast lump to be admitted to hospital and have a general anaesthetic for a biopsy of the lump. Before receiving the anaesthetic, she was warned that if the lump was found to be malignant the breast would be removed. Such a clinical approach was a psychologically stressful imposition on a patient who was already worried about the possibility of cancer. The additional stress of wondering if, on awaking from her anaesthetic, she would find her breast removed, often gave rise to many hours of silent anxiety. Fortunately, this has been recognized and nowadays many surgeons will take a different approach. They will ask you to come to the ward for day surgery, under local anaesthesia. This means that you are admitted in the morning, then be taken down to theatre where your consultant will remove all or part of your breast lump under local anaesthetic. You then return home that evening and are asked to return to see your consultant in the outpatients clinic when he has the results of the biopsy. If it is cancerous he can then discuss with you and your partner the surgical alternatives that are now open.

What will happen to me if I am told that I have breast cancer?

To be told that one has cancer – any type of cancer – is for most people, one of the worst moments of their life. They may have suspected for some time that they had cancer but had hoped that their worst fears would not have been realized.

The psychological implications of receiving the news that you have cancer is a new and extremely worrying situation. It is glib to say that you should not worry; that you should have a positive attitude towards both the diagnosis, the treatment and conquest of breast cancer. This is far easier said than done and is normally the well-intentioned advice given by those who themselves do not have cancer.

It is because I feel that all psychological aspects of cancer are so important from the moment that the diagnosis is confirmed through all stages of treatment that I have devoted a large part of the last section in this book (pp.130ff) to answering your questions about these psychological problems. The specific psychological problems of breast cancer are discussed on pp.130-135. Here I shall deal with the purely technical aspects of the treatment of breast cancer.

What types of treatment will be available to me if I am found to have breast cancer?

Having broken the news that you have cancer of the breast, your consultant will discuss the different forms of treatment which are available to you. The initial programme will normally be some form of surgery or radiotherapy, either alone or in combination. It is not possible, however, when describing surgery for breast cancer to be absolutely definitive about any one particular surgical procedure since this will depend on the stage of development of the cancer.

When talking about the staging of a cancer I described how, by looking at the microscopic make-up of the tumour cells together with the spread of these cells, your surgeon can stage the disease so that he knows how far advanced the disease process has become, and can then decide what treatment is best suited to the particular stage that the cancer has reached. There will be several treatments for the different stages of the condition. But even though surgeons may agree upon the staging of breast cancer, there is still debate as to what the best treatment is for each particular stage. I am not going to go into the pros and the cons of all the forms of surgical treatment here, but shall simply describe the more common surgical procedures, though in your own particular case your consultant will discuss the surgical approach that he is going to follow. He will be well aware that breast surgery is a very personal and highly emotive procedure for any woman to have to contemplate. Rest assured that he wants to do the best thing for you and that his advice will always be in your best interests.

What sorts of surgical procedures are there for breast cancer?

These can vary from a lumpectomy (removal of the cancerous lump) to various types of mastectomy (removal of the breast). A very common procedure is simple mastectomy followed by radiotherapy.

A modification of this operation is simple mastectomy together with the removal of lymph nodes beneath the skin in the armpit, which may be combined with a course of post-operative radiotherapy. A more extensive operation, though nowadays less commonly performed, is the radical mastectomy (mastectomy combined with removal of all the axillary lymph nodes and some of the muscular tissue upon which the breast lies).

Alternatively, there are other, less disfiguring approaches which result in the preservation of the breast appearance. For instance, the bulk of the breast tissue can be removed leaving the overlying breast skin and nipple. The space created by the removal of the breast tissue can then be filled with an artificial material called silicone to give the breast back its original shape. An even less radical operation is to simply remove the cancerous tissue within the breast, followed by radiotherapy to the remaining breast tissue and the local lymph nodes.

In a few cases where the tumour is small, showing a low degree of malignancy and no signs of spread, surgeons will advise that the cancer can be treated by radiotherapy alone. I should add, however, that this last form of treatment is controversial and is not widely practised in the UK.

Whatever the staging of your disease you will, within a few days, be admitted to hospital for treatment (see pp.38-39 for information on hospital admission procedures).

What can I expect after my operation for breast cancer?

There are several considerations to bear in mind: the immediate problems of post-operative care as well as radiotherapy, chemotherapy and hormone therapy; the all-important issues associated with breast prostheses (false breasts), breast implants, exercises, clothes, and generally adapting to a new lifestyle that a mastectomy can bring.

Let us begin by looking at what happens immediately following your operation. When you come round from the anaesthetic the first thing that you may notice will be a dressing over the site of the operation. You will probably find that you have been laid on your side and that an intravenous drip is going in to your arm. This may be a blood transfusion to correct any possibility of post-operative anaemia, or alternatively, a saline drip.

Once you are more oriented you will be propped up in bed and your blood pressure and pulse will be checked. By this time, as you become more conscious, you will almost certainly be experiencing mild discomfort from the operation site. If the discomfort borders upon pain tell the nursing staff immediately. They will be able to give you an intramuscular injection to relieve the pain.

You will also notice a small piece of rubber tubing protruding from the operating site. This is what is known as the wound drain. It is inserted by the surgeon at the time of operation and allows for the drainage of any excess tissue fluid from the operation site. This wound drain is normally removed after 24 hours.

The next day, after being assisted with a wash, you will be encouraged to sit out of bed. You may still have an intravenous drip in your arm but this early mobilization is essential for it will greatly reduce any possibility of deep vein thrombosis in your legs. It will also assist you with breathing exercises.

Sitting out of bed for a short time on the first day after your operation is normally all you will be asked to do. On your second post-operative day, if there are no contra-indications, your physiotherapist will introduce you to gentle arm and shoulder movements. These will not be too vigorous at first because the site of your operation wound will still be very much in the early stages of healing. But it is important to start some movement of the arm and shoulder as soon as possible, especially if some part of the shoulder muscle has been removed at operation. If the arm and shoulder are not mobilized fairly soon, stiffness of the shoulder joint together with muscular weakness of the arm are almost certain to occur. This may make it difficult not only to use the arm but also to move arm and shoulder in such necessary activities as washing and dressing.

At first these physiotherapy exercises will be slightly uncomfortable, but as you find your arm beginning to regain its old strength the discomfort will ease. After about a week, when it is time for you to leave hospital, you will find that your arm will be rapidly gaining its old strength and range of movements.

After my operation will I have radiotherapy?

There are no definite guidelines about radiotherapy. There is still debate as to the best forms of radiotherapy under different circumstances. In addition to this, your own particular situation – your specific form of breast cancer with its own staging – has to be considered.

Here, therefore, I shall simply describe in general terms the major types of radiotherapy that are given, one of which you will probably receive.

There is a school of thought (particularly popular in the United States) which believes that radiation to the affected breast before the operation can, by irradiating both the cancer cells within the tumour and any cancer cells that might have spread to the lymph nodes, benefit the ultimate outlook. More commonly, however, you will receive radiotherapy after your operation. (For general information about radiotherapy, see pp.45-47). This post-operative radiotherapy will be directed at the tissues in the immediate vicinity of the removed cancer as well as the lymph nodes surrounding these tissues. These lymph nodes are in the axilla, in the areas above and below the collarbone (known as the supraclavicular and infraclavicular nodes). Radiotherapy will also be directed at the lymph nodes that lie just beneath the breast-bone, known as the internal mammary nodes. Generally, 16 to 20 treatments are required, which would mean attending the radiotherapy department for four days every week for a month. This may sound a somewhat daunting exercise but after the first week you will find the visits become almost routine.

It is important to emphasize that although you may experience some minor side-effects while undergoing radiotherapy such as feeling tired or slightly sick this is normally the most you are likely to have to contend with. Side-effects will rarely be so intense as to preclude you from completing a course of radiotherapy. And remember, when you are having a course of radiotherapy you are *not* radioactive or in any way a radiation danger to your friends and family.

Radiotherapy can also be given in a different form. Radioactive needles containing a radioactive compound called irridium can be directly inserted into breast cancers. These needles deliver an exceptionally high amount of radiation that is concentrated in a very small area.

What form does chemotherapy take for breast cancer?

Chemotherapeutic drugs act by destroying rapidly dividing cells. The cells that divide most rapidly are normally cancerous cells. The theory of chemotherapy is therefore to give a drug that will reach all tissues of the body but will selectively kill only the cancerous cells. But the problem with these chemotherapeutic agents is that they can also damage normal tissues. So, in theory, although chemotherapy would appear to be the answer to selectively eliminating cancer cells, its drawback is the varying degrees of damage that it can inflict upon normal cells. It is because of this problem that the dosages of chemotherapeutic agents must be carefully balanced. On the one hand, the dosage must not be large enough to endanger the normal cells but on the other it must be adequate to fulfil its function of killing cancer cells.

It is for this reason that chemotherapy necessarily has its side-effects (see p.49) and it is important, if you are receiving chemotherapy, that you are aware of these. As soon as you notice them beginning to appear, you must tell your doctor without delay.

A course of chemotherapy normally involves the use of a combination of chemotherapeutic agents, otherwise known as cytotoxic drugs. These drugs are drawn from four main groups: alkylating agents, cytotoxic antibiotics, antimetabolites and a group of miscellaneous cytotoxic drugs. For those who want more details about specific drugs that they might be receiving I have included a detailed description of the more commonly used drugs in each of these four groups in the Drug Glossary on pp.156-159.

Some of these drugs are given by mouth, others have to be given intravenously. Combination cytotoxic therapy normally involves taking some of these drugs by mouth while also receiving others intravenously, though normally, if you are to receive an intravenous chemotherapeutic agent this will require admission to hospital either just for the day or perhaps overnight.

Before treatment starts your doctor will carry out one or more of the following tests: routine blood tests to ascertain the levels of platelets, white cells and red cells in your blood; a bone marrow biopsy, and perhaps a liver biopsy.

Chemotherapy will then be given. The procedure is painless, though side-effects may sometimes be experienced. In the vast majority of those receiving cytotoxic therapy no immediate adverse effects are seen.

When you have received your first course of cytotoxic therapy you will then reattend the outpatients clinic when blood tests will be done to assess the effectiveness of the therapy. If you are not showing any side-effects you will be given a further course of chemotherapy. Depending on how you respond to chemotherapy, treatment can continue at intervals for anything up to 12 months according to the particular combination therapy that you are being given.

What does hormone therapy for breast cancer involve?

A particular group of chemicals, called hormones, which are produced by the body's endocrine glands, are believed, in some indirect way, to have an effect on the development of some cancers. This is particularly the case in cancer of the breast. It has recently been discovered that certain breast cancers are, to some extent, dependent upon the hormone oestrogen, which is secreted by the ovary. This is not to say that breast cancer is caused by oestrogen but, rather, that oestrogen indirectly has an additive effect on the overall rate of growth of the cancer. Such cancers are referred to as being 'hormone-dependent'. The pathology laboratory, when it receives a specimen of turmour cells, can tell whether or not the tumour is responsive to the hormone oestrogen. For many years – long before it was known that some breast cancers were dependent upon oestrogen – it was realized that certain breast cancers responded to the removal of both ovaries, an operation called bilateral oophorectomy. A modification of this treatment was irradiation of the ovaries, thereby preventing them from secreting oestrogen.

Recently, advances have been made in the treatment of these oestrogen-dependent tumours without having recourse to surgery or radiotherapy. Two drugs have been found to prevent oestrogen from stimulating these tumours. If the pathology laboratory reports that a breast cancer is 'hormone-dependent' either one of these drugs will be given. One, the more commonly used, is tamoxifen, the other drug is aminoglutethmide.

They prevent hormones which are chemically related to oestrogen but which are secreted by the adrenal gland from stimulating growth in these oestrogen-responsive tumours. Due to this new form of drug treatment operations to remove the ovaries or irradiation therapy to the ovaries are now less frequently carried out in the treatment of breast cancer.

What can I do to maintain a normal general appearance following an operation on my breast?

A very important part of psychological rehabilitation is a sense of physical wellbeing, a sense that you feel and look exactly as you did before your mastectomy. It is for this reason that it is important to obtain a properly fitting breast prosthesis; to know what clothes are best worn with a prosthesis; and to be aware of and practise a range of shoulder and arm exercises.

First, breast prostheses. A breast prosthesis is a material substitute for the breast that has been removed at operation. As we have already seen, there are many different sorts of operative procedures, leaving many different forms of operative result. Consequently, many different types of prostheses are available. In general they can be divided into two groups: temporary and permanent.

When should I be fitted for a temporary breast prosthesis?

One cannot be completely dogmatic about this question because there are a number of post-operative factors that must be taken into account. For example, the skin upon which the prosthesis lies must be adequately healed.

If there have been post-operative complications such as a minor infection then this area of skin will normally take some time to settle down. If radiotherapy has been given to the operation site there may, for a time, be some form of skin reaction to this therapy.

All these factors must be taken into consideration because if the temporary prosthesis is fitted too early it can sometimes be uncomfortable to wear and may delay healing of the skin beneath.

The main aims of the temporary prosthesis are to give you back your normal breast shape while at the same time avoiding, as much as possible, any unnecessary rubbing or pressure on the scar tissue or the operation site.

Your surgeon will decide when the time is right for you to have your temporary prosthesis and will prescribe one for you. He will do this in close association with a mastectomy counsellor who is normally a nurse with special training in this field and will be able to advise you on all aspects of physical and psychological care. The prosthesis is placed in the cup of your bra and will rest gently against your chest wall (old, comfortable, soft bras are best for this). Try and avoid metal clasps on the bra straps and bras that do not have wire in the cups to support them. Sometimes the seams on bras can cause friction. Under these circumstances try turning them inside out to alleviate the problem.

When will I be able to wear my permanent breast prosthesis?

When the operation site is fully healed, you will be able to get your permanent prosthesis. Now, to be quite frank, in this area there is a problem.

Most experts will tell you that the best permanent prostheses are those made of silicone. There are many advantages to silicone prostheses, which are as follows: they look very natural and can be worn under any clothing and also, to a certain extent, swimwear; the silicone itself has a consistency remarkably like breast tissue and, to all intents and purposes, feels very similar to a real breast (this is why many cosmetic surgeons actually use silicone implants for breast augmentation procedures); they don't need to be worn inside bras; they will absorb heat from your body wall and so will gain body temperature. Also, silicone as a material is very resistant to damage. If, for example, you are using it with a swimsuit it will not be affected by water – even seawater – and, if for any reason it is either cut or punctured, the silicone contents will not leak away.

However, there is one major drawback to silicone prostheses – cost. Theoretically, they are available under the National Health Service, but sometimes they are very difficult to get. It is true that whatever the consultant puts on his prescription can, in theory, be obtained from the hospital appliances department. But, unfortunately, in some hospitals this is simply not the case. If you *are* unable to obtain a silicone prosthesis on the National Health, therefore, you may feel that it is worth your while to buy your own and many women are forced to do this.

You can, of course, have more than one prosthesis. Even temporary prostheses can be used now and again because they are very light and, because of this, very comfortable.

If you are given a prosthesis that does not seem to suit you don't just accept it; explain its drawbacks to your consultant or your mastectomy counsellor. Under these circumstances you will always get a sympathetic ear and should eventually get the prosthesis that is best suited to your particular needs.

What sort of clothes should I wear?

This should not present too much in the way of problems because radical mastectomy is an operation that is going out of vogue. In the past it was this operation that used to present the most post-operative cosmetic problems for in some circumstances it involved the removal of variable amounts of muscular tissue in and around the armpit and the chest wall. This led to a deficiency of tissue that was in some cases difficult to hide.

But even following a simple mastectomy the features of your upper arm and chest wall may noticeably be changed. This may mean you having to think about clothes with higher necklines than you might normally wear and also tops with sleeves that are long enough to cover up any unsightly areas of which you may be self-conscious.

Sometimes, instead of wearing a bra with a prosthesis inserted into one of the cups it may be possible to adapt a dress with a small pocket that will take a prosthesis. This type of adaptation is particularly useful for summer wear when some prostheses can become slightly prickly in very hot or humid conditions. In most cases, either adapting or buying new clothes will cope with the situation and most problems of appearance can be overcome.

The one area where many women do find a problem, however, is with swimwear. Very few manufacturers design and make swimwear specifically for women who have had mastectomies. Prostheses can be worn with ordinary swimwear but some, especially those that absorb water, do have their limitations, and this is where the silicone prostheses are so useful.

If you look to the end of this book (pp. 160) you will see that I have given, in the section of Useful Addresses, the names of associations to whom you can write and who will send you brochures and helpful hints on clothes and swimwear especially designed for women who have had a mastectomy.

Are there any exercises that I should do after my mastectomy?

After your mastectomy, both the nurses on the ward and the physio-therapist will show you how to gradually mobilize your arm with a series of graded exercises. When you go home it is important that you do not allow your arm and shoulder joint to stiffen up and it is a good idea to do daily exercises for at least a month following discharge from hospital. Before you do these, however, do consult your doctor to make sure that he agrees with them.

Here are just a few of the exercises that you might like to try. Face a wall and put both your palms on the wall. Then, alternately, lift each hand away from the wall and place it six inches or so above where it was – rather like 'walking up the wall'. The effect of this exercise is to stretch both your arms and shoulder joints. Alternatively, while sitting down, try clasping your hands behind your head and gently rotating your shoulders from side to side. You will find another excellent form of exercise is swimming.

When doing ordinary household tasks, do not try to protect the affected arm and shoulder but, conversely, try and use them rather more than you would otherwise do. When vacuum cleaning, for example, push the cleaner with the affected arm rather than the good arm. In this way household chores can be combined with exercise. Similarly, if polishing, try and get the arm and shoulder of the operation side into action.

The basic message in all these movements is to get the operated arm and shoulder into action. Don't overdo it. The exercises shouldn't actually cause any pain, but a certain amount of discomfort will mean that they are doing you some good.

What is lymphoedema of the arm?

This is an uncommon complication following some mastectomy operations. It is uniform swelling of the arm which can occur from any time following the operation and in some cases may occur years later. Lymphoedema used to be seen much more commonly when radical mastectomy was the operation of choice for breast cancer. As this operation is now being done less often, it is less commonly seen. If you do get lymphoedema of the arm, your doctor will supervise the treatment.

You will be advised to raise the affected arm as much as possible, especially when you are not using it. For instance, when you are sitting down it can be rested on a raised soft cushion. Similarly, while you are sleeping it can be elevated on a pillow.

Using the swollen arm can usually reduce the swelling, as will wearing elastic sleeves especially designed for this purpose. Alternatively your doctor may refer you to your local physiotherapy department, where the physiotherapist will arrange for you to have a series of exercises designed to reduce the swelling. In certain circumstances a compressive sleeve pump can also be applied to your arm, under strict supervision, and the fluid painlessly forced out of the arm.

One important thing to remember is that, with lymphoedema of the arm, the arm is particularly prone to infection so be sure to protect your arm at all times. For instance, if you are working in the garden, always wear gloves. If you think that your arm or even a finger is showing signs of infection, report this to your doctor immediately because infections in arms with lymphoedema can be a serious problem.

What is lung cancer?

Lung cancer is a blanket term, referring to any cancer arising in the lung, but is no more specific than this. There are in fact about eight different major cancers that arise in the lung and some of these are sub-divided into more specialized cancers. As lung cancer is such a common cancer I shall mention four of the most common types. Although lung cancer is a serious condition it is worth emphasizing that some of these cancers have a better outlook than others, and are, in fact, eminently treatable.

The commonest type of lung cancer is known as squamous cell carcinoma, and is found most commonly in smokers. Although squamous cell carcinomas grow very rapidly, in certain circumstances they are less likely to spread than other lung cancers. Another type, known as the adenocarcinoma, occurs proportionately in both smokers and non-smokers and may spread rather more easily than the squamous carcinoma. The third major type is known as the anaplastic small cell carcinoma. When seen under the microscope this cancer is said to resemble clumps of oatcells – hence its alternative name, oatcell carcinoma. This form of lung cancer is very malignant and can spread rapidly throughout the body. It is, in fact, often at the sites of spread that the first signs of this cancer are seen. The fourth major type of lung cancers are known as the anaplastic large cell carcinomas. Like the oatcell cancers, these are extremely malignant, the main difference between them being the different approaches to their treatment.

Although the four major forms of lung cancers which I have just mentioned make up by far and away the majority of lung cancers seen there is also another important type known as mesothelioma. It is of importance because it is caused by asbestos, and is one of the few cancers of which we definitely know the cause. Not only does this make this type of cancer amenable to prevention, but it also provides a useful starting point for research into lung cancer in general.

What causes lung cancer?

Everybody, or nearly everybody, knows that cigarette-smoking can cause lung cancer. What is not generally known is that this was only recently proved. It was the pioneering work of the epidemiologist Sir Richard Doll in the 1950s and 1960s that was able to establish the definitive and conclusive link between cigarette-smoking and lung cancer.

The carcinogen responsible for causing lung cancer almost certainly lies in the tar content of inhaled cigarette smoke, although its exact identity still remains a mystery. This is why the tar content of cigarettes is so widely advertised. However, this advertising gives the distinctly incorrect impression that low-tar cigarettes are safe. True, low-tar cigarettes are safer than high-tar cigarettes, but low-tar cigarettes are still lethal themselves.

The message is quite simple. By smoking cigarettes you are killing yourself. The only difference between high-tar cigarettes and low-tar cigarettes is that with the high-tar varieties you are killing yourself more quickly.

Many other subtle advertising messages and rumours are quite without foundation. It is, for example, often suggested that smokers who inhale are at a greater risk than those who do not. There is no proof to support this assumption. Inhalers and exhalers are all equally at risk. It is also stated that pipe-smokers and cigar-smokers are less at risk than cigarette-smokers, but evidence for this is scanty. However, there are encouraging statistics. For example, if you have just taken up smoking and you give up smoking today your chances of developing the disease are virtually nil.

When Sir Richard Doll first discovered that cigarette-smoking was related to lung cancer, he encouraged a large number of doctors to give up smoking.

When he compared the doctors who had given up smoking to a similar group of doctors who had *not* given up smoking he was able to show quite conclusively that those doctors who had given up smoking were far less likely to develop the disease than those who had not. In other words, even if you have smoked for a long time, giving up smoking today may well save your life, in the long term.

Originally, lung cancer was predominantly a disease of men, the problem being rarely seen in women. But as women have adopted the habit of smoking, lung cancer is being seen more frequently in the female population.

However, not all lung cancer is due to smoking. As I have said, one type can definitely be attributed to asbestos, and there are other industrial processes that are known to cause the disease – most specifically in the chrome and nickel ore industries.

It is also believed that some lung cancers may develop from chronic lung infection. Most chronic bronchitics are smokers, however, and in such cases it is difficult to know how much the cancer has been caused by the effects of the chronic bronchitis and how much by the carcinogens in the tar fraction in the inhaled cigarette smoke. The bottom line, however, is this: *Smoking causes lung cancer.*

What are the symptoms of lung cancers?

Cancer of the lung is a disease which has no really specific symptoms, as such. It is important if you are in a high risk group for lung cancer – in other words, if you are a smoker – that if you notice either one or more of the following symptoms, you see your doctor.

The symptoms of lung cancer fall into two major groups. The first is concerned directly with the chest; the second is a somewhat more nebulous collection of symptoms but ones which should be taken seriously in the high-risk group of smokers.

Symptoms relating to the chest are by far and away the most common, but one of the problems with making a diagnosis of lung cancer on the basis of these chest symptoms is that they are very easily confused with the symptoms of chronic bronchitis – namely, chronic, rasping coughing together with the bringing up of sputum (phlegm/spit) and varying grades and degrees of breathlessness together with bouts of chest pain. There may also be feelings of tightness in the chest, together with a noticeable wheezing sound or sensation, especially when exercise is taken or in cold weather. Both you and your doctor need to decide whether these symptoms are just simply those of ongoing chronic bronchitis or the symptoms of lung cancer. The problem is that in many cases one simply cannot tell the difference.

However, there is one most important sign that must never be ignored and should be reported to your doctor, immediately. This is blood in the sputum – a condition known as haemoptysis. Even if you see faint specks of blood in your sputum these warning signs must not be ignored. Another very important warning sign, whether or not you are a chronic bronchitic, is a lack of improvement after a bad cold, a bad bout of influenza or even a bout of pneumonia. If the chronic infection appears to be lingering for longer than normal, report this fact to your doctor. As a chronic bronchitic, you will know when your 'normal' chronic bronchitic state appears, in some way, to be changing for the worse.

And so to the other broad group of symptoms. Some of these are the general symptoms that accompany so many cancerous and non-cancerous diseases. They include loss of appetite and weight, as well as a general slowing down, a feeling that you cannot do the tasks that you used to be able to do perfectly well.

In very rare cases, lung cancer can arise as a muscular weakness or diseases caused by hormonal overproduction such as thyrotoxicosis or Cushing's disease. Some lung cancers are detected on routine chest X-ray in an otherwise symptomless patient.

The essential point is this. If you are a cigarette-smoker who has smoked cigarettes for some time and notice any of the above symptoms, or anything that makes you think that you are not 'quite right' and the symptoms persist, do not just assume that they are going to go away. Go and see your doctor and get a full check-up.

What tests am I likely to have if lung cancer is suspected?

Before any tests are done you will have a full physical examination, though, in the majority of patients with lung cancer, this often reveals no outward signs of lung cancer. Sometimes, if the cancer is at an advanced stage, your doctor will be able to hear sounds of an obstruction in your chest with a stethoscope. By percussing your chest he may be able to outline fluid on the lung known as a pleural infusion. By feeling deep into the base of your neck he may also be able to identify hard lymph nodes that have been invaded by spreading cancer cells. Similarly, by feeling your abdomen, and particularly the area over the liver, he might detect a liver enlargement which could be due to a secondary spread of the cancer. A routine blood test will also be done to see whether or not you are anaemic.

Often the examination will throw up nothing in the way of a positive diagnosis. Your doctor will then proceed to a series of tests. The first and probably the most important is the chest X-ray. The majority of lung cancers will show up by this procedure. In certain cases the radiologist, on looking at the X-ray, may still be unsure as to whether it demonstrates definitive evidence of cancer. Under such circumstances he will ask for a further series of more specialized X-rays known as tomograms. These are very useful in differentiating cancerous growths from other lesions. Alternatively, he may order a CAT scan (see p.35) to establish the diagnosis.

Apart from these X-ray tests you will be asked to provide a sputum specimen. This will allow the pathologist to look for evidence of malignant cells; the technique is known as sputum cytology.

Following these investigations, which are normally done on an out-patient basis, if the diagnosis of lung cancer is a possibility you will be asked to come back to the hospital for further tests. These too are usually conducted on an outpatient basis though you may be asked to stay over-night. The most common and most important of these specialized tests is bronchoscopy. In this procedure the consultant will pass a fibre-optiscope (see p.32) down your trachea (windpipe) and into your lungs. This will allow him to directly visualize the inside of your lungs and specifically the main bronchi. He will already have some idea where he needs to look, from the chest X-ray, and so will direct the fibre-optiscope along the bronchi until he can see the suspicious area that was outlined on the X-ray. By looking at the lesion directly, he will probably be able to establish whether or not it is cancer. He can also take a biopsy from the lesion, using a small biopsy unit incorporated in the fibre-opticscope. This biopsy will then be sent to the laboratory so that the precise form of lung cancer can be established – an important consideration when deciding upon treatment.

In addition to the bronchoscopy a further investigation called a mediastinoscopy may be needed. In this procedure a fibre-optiscope is passed into the top of the chest, allowing the surgeon to look at the outer aspects of the air passages, together with the lymph nodes surrounding these air passages. In this way, any spread of the cancer to the lymph nodes can be detected. If these nodes have already been infiltrated by cancer, then surgery will probably not be advised.

If it is felt that the cancer may have spread to other parts of the body, radio-isotope scanning can be carried out to establish whether or not metastases have reached the bones or the liver. It is important to know this in planning long-term treatment. Sometimes the cancer can spread from the lung to the brain. If such a spread is suspected, a CAT scan may be needed as a further investigation.

Am I likely to have an operation for my lung cancer?

There are three forms of treatment for lung cancer: surgery, radiotherapy and chemotherapy. The most successful treatment, in terms of cure, is surgery. However, certain lung cancers are not amenable to surgery. This may be because they are too advanced by the time they are discovered. Alternatively the original cancer itself might be small, but it may have spread to distant parts of the body.

The decision as to whether or not you should undergo surgery will necessarily depend on a number of factors which the results of your investigations will have thrown up. It is difficult to be dogmatic because no two cases are exactly the same but, in general terms, if your consultant feels that there is a good chance of effecting a cure by surgery then this initial procedure will be advised. Earlier, I mentioned specific forms of lung cancer. Two of these – adenocarcinoma and the squamous cell carcinoma – are the forms of lung cancer that are most amenable to surgery. About half the patients who are diagnosed as suffering from these forms of lung cancers will be offered surgery as the primary procedure. If, however, the spread of these cancers appears to be extensive at the time of diagnosis surgery is not always the preferred solution. In the case of oatcell lung cancer, unless this tumour is very small at the time of diagnosis and there is no evidence of spread, surgery is not normally recommended.

What does surgery for lung cancer involve?

The operation involves the surgeon opening up the chest under a general anaesthetic and removing the diseased part of the lung, together with any lymph nodes that appear to have been affected by the spreading cancer. It may seem extraordinary but even though half your lung may be removed, the remaining half will more than adequately cope with your respiratory needs. Apart from occasional long-term breathlessness, the loss of half a lung is barely noticed.

When you come around from the anaesthetic you may find tubes coming out of your chest wall. These are known as chest drains, and have two purposes. One is to drain away unwanted secretions and blood that may have accumulated at the operation site. The other is to allow the part of the lung that has been left behind to expand normally.

In my earlier accounts of the post-operative phase, I mentioned that physiotherapy is always an important aspect of care. In post-operative chest cases, it is particularly important and one of the first things that the physiotherapist will teach you will be breathing exercises. Sometimes you may even be taught these exercises before the operation in preparation for the post-operative phase.

One of the major problems after any chest operation is that secretions tend to accumulate in the lungs. Because of this a very important part of your post-operative physiotherapy will be postural drainage. This involves being positioned in such a way as to allow the accumulated secretions to run out of your lungs. To assist this your physiotherapist will gently percuss your chest wall with her hands with due care and attention to the operative site.

While the remaining lung is recovering, you may be given oxygen therapy by mask. Some patients are attached to an artificial respirator to assist breathing. This is a painless procedure, but does require a certain amount of sedation. As I have said, you will be surprised at how soon your breathing gets back to normal after the operation, and most patients are discharged a week to ten days later.

Will I be given radiotherapy?

Most patients with lung cancer receive radiotherapy. This includes both patients who have had an operation and those for whom surgery was not appropriate. Particular care must be taken with patients who have not undergone surgery, however, since larger doses of radiotherapy will need to be given.

Radiotherapy can sometimes be a strain on someone who is elderly and not in the best of general health. This is why it is so important to check that the patient is in the best physical state possible before a course of radiotherapy is begun.

For example, with a high-protein diet which may include special milk supplements the patient's strength should be built up.

Radiotherapy for lung cancer is the same as for other types of cancer (see pp.45-47). There will almost certainly be side-effects which include a general feeling of tiredness, lack of appetite and, in some cases, nausea and sickness. Treatment will normally be carried out on an outpatient basis and will be given in daily treatments extending over a period of four to six weeks. As well as being directed at the primary lung cancer, radiotherapy is often given to treat metastases, particularly those that have spread to the bones and the brain. This has the effect of reducing the size of secondary cancers as well as reducing the pain that they can sometimes cause.

What does chemotherapy for lung cancer involve?

Chemotherapy is often given as additional therapy following operation and radiotherapy. It may be given orally, by intravenous injection, or intravenous infusion (for general information on chemotherapy, see pp.48-51).

Chemotherapy can be a particularly effective form of treatment for patients with oatcell cancer, for whom surgery is not normally undertaken. As well as being effective in varying degrees for the other forms of lung cancer, it is also a useful treatment for metastases, particularly when it is used in conjunction with radiotherapy.

Chemotherapy for lung cancer is normally given in what is known as combination therapy, meaning that a number of drugs are given simultaneously – though not necessarily all at the same time – resulting in a cumulative effect.

Commonly used drugs for lung cancer are adriamycin, cyclophosphamide, vincristine and etoposide.

What are the long-term problems of lung cancer?

These problems can broadly be divided into two groups: those connected with the chest and breathing and those connected with the spread of the cancer.

One of the commonest and most troublesome local effects of lung cancer is known as a pleural effusion. This is accumulation of fluid on the lung. The fluid does not actually enter the lung but, by occupying part of the lung cavity, prevents the lung from expanding, so making breathing difficult. If weeks, months, or even years following an operation for lung cancer you find that you are getting breathing difficulties report this problem to your doctor. If you are having routine outpatient follow-up appointments, however, the condition will probably be spotted on a chest X-ray before it gives marked breathing difficulties.

Pleural effusions are treated as follows. You will be admitted to hospital on an outpatient basis. Once in the ward you will be placed in a sitting position either in a chair or in bed. A local anaesthetic will then be applied to your chest wall and a syringe will be passed painlessly through the chest wall and into the area of lung in which the fluid has accumulated. The fluid can then be drawn off with an immediate relief to your breathing problems.

Lung cancer may cause problems as a result of a spread to other parts of the body. General problems following primary lung cancer result in the spread of the cancer to the brain, liver and bones. Such a spread is not necessarily painful but, if pain *is* a problem, then radiotherapy and chemotherapy as well as the liberal use of pain-killing drugs will normally relieve it.

What is bowel cancer?

When a surgeon actually opens up the bowel and looks at the site of a bowel cancer it can be seen to take two distinct forms. It may be seen as an ulcerated area growing into the wall of the bowel, or it can take the form of an ulcerated polyp – a balloon-like structure – growing from the wall of the bowel. It is by looking at these particular forms of growth and the depth of their spread into the bowel wall that the staging (assessment of the degree of malignancy) can be established.

What causes bowel cancer?

With the vast majority of cancers, there may be various hints and suspicions as to their causes, but, apart from a few, rare cancers, the precise initiating factors remain an enigma. Cancer of the bowel (the colon and rectum), is no exception. However, a number of interesting facts have emerged, which will probably lead to the eventual discovery of the causes of cancer of the bowel.

One of the main culprits is believed to be diet. The first evidence for this came from the observation that bowel cancer is seen much more commonly in Western societies than in the African subcontinent.

There are distinct differences in the diets of these populations. In Western societies diet consists mainly of high levels of fat and animal protein with a relatively low fibre content. Carbohydrate, in these diets, is also refined. Conversely, in African societies, the diet is high in fibre, high in unrefined carbohydrates and low in both animal fat and animal protein. However, it is not these particular dietary constituents that are thought to be at fault in themselves but, rather, the effect that they have upon the passage of foods through the bowel itself. The high fibre content of non-Western diets increases the food bulk, and consequently the residue, that makes up the bowel content. The qualities of a softer consistency, together with greater bulk allow for a more rapid passage of the faeces through the large bowel. Conversely, the Western-style diet results in smaller and harder faeces which tend to pass through the bowel more slowly. The dietary theory of bowel cancer suggests that the faeces contain substances which cause cancer (known as carcinogens) and that because these carcinogens tend to remain for a longer time, and in a more concentrated form, against the innermost layer of the bowel wall (known as the mucosa) cancer is more likely to develop there.

Searches have been made for these carcinogenic substances in the faeces. The prime suspect at the time of writing would appear to be bile salts, although another is a bacterium called bacteroides which is found in high levels in populations that are particularly prone to developing bowel cancer. Interestingly, when a race such as the Japanese are uprooted by migration to Western society, the incidence of bowel cancer, which is normally very low in Japan, rises rapidly as they adopt the American diet.

Is diet the only possible cause of bowel cancer?

There are a number of factors which make an individual more likely to develop bowel cancer. The first of these is a general genetic predisposition.

The incidence of bowel cancer appears to be greater in those families in whom bowel cancer has appeared in previous generations. This not to say that bowel cancer is inherited, though there are rare forms of inherited bowel disease that can lead on to the disease. An example is familial polyposis, in which numerous polyps develop in the wall of the bowel. Eventually some of these polyps may develop into bowel cancer.

Another non-cancerous condition that can develop into bowel cancer is ulcerative colitis (a chronic inflammation of the bowel wall), though I must emphasize that only about 5 per cent of those suffering with ulcerative colitis are at risk. In addition, that 5 per cent will be suffering with the most severe form of ulcerative colitis, and only a small proportion of this number may go on to develop bowel cancer.

What are the symptoms of bowel cancer?

Before answering this, it may be useful to describe the bowel itself. Anatomically, the bowel, or large intestine, arises on the right side of the abdomen as a structure known as the caecum. It travels up and across the right side of the abdomen where it is referred to as the ascending and transverse colon. The remaining part of the large bowel travels down the left-hand side of the abdomen, exiting at the anus. The parts of this section of the large bowel are the descending colon, the sigmoid colon and the rectum.

The symptoms of bowel cancer can fall into two main groups: those from the right side of the large bowel and those from the left.

As with most cancers, it is important to remember, however, that symptoms are only general indicators and not specific signposts for cancer. Just because you have one or more of the following abdominal symptoms, therefore, does not mean that you automatically have cancer.

On the other hand, do not ignore them altogether. If you are experiencing an abdominal symptom for the first time and it is not what might be termed 'normal' for you, then it is important that you consult your doctor.

Symptoms of cancers arising from the right side of the large bowel tend to be somewhat indefinite in nature. There may be intermittent changes of bowel habit, and a slight loss of weight and appetite. People may say that you are looking rather paler than usual. When your GP examines you he may find nothing or perhaps just a vague mass on the right side of your abdomen.

Symptoms of cancers arising from the left side of the abdomen, are usually more definite in nature. You may, for example, notice a change in your bowel habit which lasts over a period of weeks. A person with normally loose stools may notice that constipation may become a problem. Conversely, someone who normally suffers with constipation may notice that their motions are looser and more frequent than usual. Some patients also describe spasmodic pain, particularly in the lower left part of the abdomen. Others describe feelings of lower abdominal fullness, together with a sensation of inability to evacuate their bowel. Such symptoms should never be ignored, especially if you do not normally have them.

One symptom that should never be ignored is blood in the stools. Even if there is the smallest speck, you must report it to your doctor. Do not automatically assume though that you have cancer of the bowel. There are many harmless, non-cancerous causes for this symptom. One very common cause is haemorrhoids, or piles; another is diverticulitis. Even if you had either of these conditions diagnosed in the past, however, you must still check with your doctor. Don't simply assume that the bleeding is a recurrence of a former condition.

Sometimes bowel cancer can reveal itself as an acute intestinal obstruction and this is very much a surgical emergency. There is invariably abdominal pain, nausea and vomiting together with complete constipation. Such a problem will require immediate hospital admission.

How will my bowel problem be investigated?

At the initial visit to your GP an examination of your abdomen, anus and rectum will be made. During the examination, your doctor will be looking for evidence of a mass in your abdomen together with any liver enlargement. He will examine your back passage to see if he can feel a growth in your rectum, and will also look for other problems in the rectum and anus, such as haemorrhoids or diverticulitis. Just because you have haemorrhoids (or any bowel condition) will not necessarily mean that you are free of bowel cancer. One of the main pitfalls in diagnosing medical problems is to assume that there is only one problem with any one particular organ. That is why doctors, if the symptoms you describe are similar to those I have mentioned above, may refer you to a hospital for further investigations.

In the past, referrals were made directly to a surgeon but now there are doctors who specialize in diseases of the gastro-intestinal tract (known as gastro-enterologists). If, following their investigations, they feel that a surgical opinion is needed, it is they who will refer you on to the surgeon. Alternatively, you may be referred directly to a surgeon. But remember, if this happens, it will not necessarily mean that you have cancer.

At your first visit to the gastro-enterologist he will once more go over the ground covered by your own doctor. He will then probably carry out a further examination, known as sigmoidoscopy. This involves passing a sigmoidoscope (a thin metal tube) through the anal sphincter, up into the rectum and sigmoid colon. There is an internal light source in the tube, which allows the gastro-enterologist to observe the mucosa (inner lining of the bowel wall). As the sigmoidoscope is gently passed up the bowel, any suspicious areas of the mucosa are noted and, if necessary, a biopsy is taken. The procedure is painless, though a slight amount of lower abdominal discomfort may be experienced for an hour or two afterwards.

There is, however, a limit to how far the gastro-enterologist can pass the sigmoidoscope up into the bowel. In order to explore both the left side of the large bowel and the transverse colon, therefore, he may go on to a procedure known as colonoscopy. The colonoscope is a solid tube composed of fibre-optic fibres, the properties of which allow light to be bent around corners. Unlike sigmoidoscopy, which can be performed without bowel preparation, a colonoscopy requires that your bowel is as free of contents as possible. This will mean your taking laxatives prescribed by your doctor for a day or two before the test. The test itself is done very much in the same manner as a sigmoidoscopy except that the instrument is passed further along the bowel.

The gastro-enterologist inspects the mucosa in this part of the bowel. If he sees any suspicious-looking areas of the mucosa, he can photograph them, and, if necessary, take a small biopsy. On removal of the colonoscope, there will be a mild sensation of lower abdominal discomfort, but no other side-effects are normally noticed.

Under certain circumstances, further examinations may be required, the most common of which is a barium enema. The object of this examination is to outline the bowel wall, using barium, a radio-opaque substance. By looking for irregularities in this outline, the radiologist will be able to determine whether or not a suspicious lesion is present. In order to complete this test successfully the bowel has to be specially prepared. Your doctor will give you a laxative together with instructions about what you must do in preparation for the barium enema.

In the radiology department you will normally be given an ordinary enema before the barium enema. The purpose of this is to wash out any residual material that may still be in your bowel. You will then be given the barium enema. This is administered by a tube that is passed through the anal sphincter into the rectum. When the enema has been introduced, X-ray pictures will be taken of your abdomen.

You will be placed in different positions, during this examination, so that different views of the bowel may be taken. When the investigation is over, the barium enema is washed out of the bowel. Lower abdominal discomfort may be experienced and, for a day or two after the examination, your stools will contain residue of the enema. Apart from these minor problems, however, there are no long-term side-effects.

Once these investigations are over, if bowel cancer is diagnosed you will be referred to a consultant surgeon who will discuss with you the best surgical approach for treating the cancer.

How is bowel cancer treated?

In many cases, cancer of the bowel is completely curable. The reason for this is that surgery can remove the tumour completely, if it is caught at an early stage. Bowel cancer is a good example of a cancer that is particularly amenable to surgery. Radiotherapy and chemotherapy may be given following surgery but are often not required because surgery is so successful.

The precise form of surgery that will be carried out will depend very much upon where the cancer is growing in your bowel. Another consideration that has to be taken into account is the speed of onset of your symptoms, and complications that might arise from the acute obstructive problems that cancer of the bowel can sometimes give.

Let us begin by considering a cancer that is affecting the right side of the bowel, together with that part of the bowel that traverses the upper part of the abdomen and some of the bowel that begins to descend down the left-hand side of the abdomen. (Technically these parts of the large bowel are known as the caecum, the ascending colon, the transverse colon and the first part of the descending colon.) Let us assume that the cancer has been discovered early and that there are no complications such as obstruction. Under these circumstances, during the operation your surgeon will take out the cancerous piece of bowel together with a variable amount of healthy bowel on either side of the cancer. Although the bowel on either side of the cancerous area may look healthy, microscopic spread of the cancer can occur and if a piece of bowel is left behind in which microscopic spread of the cancer has taken place, such a spread may cause a recurrence of the primary cancer.

Once your surgeon is satisfied that he has removed the cancer he will join the two ends of the cut bowel together (a procedure known as an anastomosis). After your operation you will find that, as the days progress, your bowels will return to complete normality. You will notice no other effects from the operation, apart from a scar on your abdomen.

For the first few days after the operation you will not be allowed to take anything by mouth. This is because abdominal operations have the effect of disturbing the rhythmic contractions of the muscles in the bowel wall. If either food or drink is taken too early, these muscles can go into spasm and a condition called paralytic ileus can result. It is to avoid this problem that, on their ward rounds, your doctors will listen to your abdomen with their stethoscopes for what are known as 'return of bowel sounds'. Once these sounds are clearly heard you will be able to resume drinking and eating, although only gradually to begin with. The other obvious reason for not eating straight after your operation is that any food passing through the bowel may cause a weakness or even a break in the anastomosis of the bowel.

Now let us take a second situation where the cancer has occurred in the left-hand side of the bowel.

The cancerous area cannot simply be removed and the two ends of the healthy bowel joined together as with the previous case. This is because, since the affected area is so near the anus, the patient would lose control over his anal sphincter. Faecal incontinence would invariably result, a feature which is obviously socially unacceptable and distressing for the patient. The other problem is that when bowel cancer arises near the anus the surgeon can never be sure that the piece of bowel lying between the cancer and the anal region is not infiltrated with cancer. It is for these reasons that a colostomy is often advised.

A colostomy is produced by bringing the open end of the large bowel to the surface through a hole in the abdominal wall known as a stoma. A colostomy is fashioned as follows. At the operation, the piece of bowel containing the cancer together with the bowel that extends to the anal region is completely removed. The anal sphincter is then closed and becomes functionless. But the bowel still has to pass faeculent waste matter, and since this matter can no longer be excreted at the anus an artificial passage has to be created. So the surgeon fashions a small round hole in the abdominal wall; the healthy end of the bowel is then passed through this hole so that the bowel contents can pass to the exterior, so creating an artifical opening on the abdominal surface.

At this stage, I should also like to mention a third surgical procedure which sometimes has to be performed in cases of bowel cancer where the cancer has either caused an acute obstruction or has caused the bowel wall to perforate. Under these circumstances an abdominal operation known as laparotomy is required. In such a situation, even though the area of bowel cancer may be on the right side of the abdomen a temporary colostomy will be required to overcome the acute surgical problem. In the operation, the primary bowel cancer is removed but instead of the two ends of free bowel being joined together, they are both brought through the abdominal wall to form the temporary colostomy. This is merely the first stage of the operation, however. Once you have sufficiently recovered (the period of recovery will vary from patient to patient) you will undergo a second abdominal operation, in which the two pieces of bowel will be joined together and replaced in your abdomen. You will therefore not be left with a permanent colostomy.

Will I have radiotherapy for bowel cancer?

Radiotherapy (see p.45) is used to treat bowel cancer, but only in conjunction with surgery. It is used mainly for those cancers which occur in the bowel on the left side of the abdomen, including cancers of the sigmoid colon and the rectum. Radiotherapy for rectal cancer can be given either before or after the operation. If it is given before the operation, about a month has to pass before you can undergo surgery in order to allow the irradiated tissues to settle down. Radiotherapy given after the operation is only given when the bowel and abdominal incision have completely healed.

What will happen after my colostomy operation?

When you come round from the operation you will probably not see the colostomy itself immediately. This is because, at the conclusion of the operation, your surgeon will have placed a bag over the abdominal area where the stoma has been sited. The first time that you will probably see your colostomy will be when the nurse comes to replace the colostomy bag. Subsequently, your stoma care therapist will take you through all aspects of colostomy care, both during your stay in hospital and after your discharge.

There are two basic approaches to colostomy care, and a combination of both may be advised. Whatever the case, this care is a very individual problem and you should be guided by your surgeon and stoma care therapist as to which is best suited to your needs.

The first and most common procedure involves using a colostomy bag to collect intestinal waste matter. Alternatively, the colostomy can be irrigated without requiring the use of a bag. I must emphasize, however, that irrigation should only be undertaken with the express consent of your consultant and following a successful period of training in colostomy irrigation technique by your stoma therapist. The reason for this is that certain bowel conditions preclude irrigation of the colostomy and might exacerbate the intestinal problem.

What does colostomy irrigation entail?

In essence, irrigation involves the following: A catheter is inserted into the colostomy. A variable amount of warm water is then passed through the catheter into the bowel, so encouraging the bowel to evacuate itself. The catheter is then removed and a piece of drainage tubing is placed over the colostomy, the other end being placed in the lavatory pan, so allowing the material to be disposed of. Having completed the irrigation and carefully wiped the skin around the colostomy (as instructed by your stoma care therapist) a cap or colostomy bag is placed over the stoma. This will catch any material that may ooze out of the colostomy, though with irrigation this is not normally a problem.

Irrigation must normally be done every 24 to 48 hours. It can take anything from 30 minutes to an hour to perform, and a pre-arranged time in the day will have to be set aside for the purpose.

Your stoma care therapist will discuss this with you and advise you where necessary once you get home.

Finally, discuss the situation with your family, and make sure they are aware about what having a colostomy means, especially as regards your having to occupy the bathroom for perhaps up to an hour at a time.

What problems will a colostomy pose?

The idea of having to cope with a colostomy is quite naturally very worrying, and may cause a great deal of anxiety.

There are many misconceptions about colostomies and what it means to have one. A lot of these worries arise from problems that were very real in the past but which, with modern techniques, have to a large extent been eliminated. In the past, little knowledge existed about the long-term care of a colostomy and there was no one to whom the patient could turn for advice. Now, not only is there a large body of knowledge which supports improved technology in caring for colostomies but there are also a number of specialized nurses who are trained to help colostomy patients in all aspects of colostomy care. These nurses are clinical specialists known as stoma care therapists.

There are also associations of patients with colostomies which are very supportive and can give much-needed advice on all aspects of long-term problems that can occur (see Useful Addresses, p.160).

You will, at some stage, be visited by a stoma care therapist. This will be before your operation. If there is enough time, the meeting can sometimes be conducted at your home. In this pre-operative visit, the stoma care therapist will describe to you what having a colostomy entails, and how you should care for your colostomy after the operation. She will also discuss the changes in lifestyle that a colostomy may bring about for you and your family. During your meeting, she may also introduce you to another patient who has had a colostomy. This exchange of information before your operation can reduce much of the worry and uncertainty that can surround fears for the future. Following your operation the stoma care therapist will be very much at your side advising and helping where necessary, as the post-operative phase evolves.

The problems of having a colostomy are predictable and never insurmountable but I cannot emphasize enough how useful it is to speak to someone who has had a colostomy for some time. Such people abound with practical hints and tips and can also psychologically encourage you to overcome many of the initial doubts and worries that quite naturally go with having to cope with a new colostomy.

Take diet, for instance. Normally a colostomy will not mean any change in diet. However, you might find that certain foods that you were used to before are not particularly well tolerated by your colostomy. Discovering what these are is inevitably a process of trial and error.

One particular problem that some patients experience is gaseous discharge from the colostomy. This is often due to foods such as baked beans and vegetables such as spinach. If you have this problem, therefore, these foods are probably best avoided.

Sometimes the skin around the colostomy can become slightly red and raw. If this problem arises, contact your stoma care therapist immediately – it may turn into a chronic skin problem unless treated quickly and effectively.

Finally, a word about the psycho-social aspects of having a colostomy. I cannot emphasize too strongly that with modern colostomy equipment there is rarely any social problem. Leakage and gaseous discharge, for example, can normally be well contained with modern stoma bags.

As far as the family is concerned, counselling by the stoma care therapist is very important. If the potential difficulties associated with stoma care are fully appreciated by all members of the family an understanding of the problem will, in a short space of time, remove the problem altogether.

What are cancer of the uterus and cervical cancer?

It is important to understand what is meant by cancer of the uterus, since the term can cover a number of different conditions which are sometimes confused. Let us consider the uterus itself. The uterus, also known as the womb, is a pear-shaped structure lying in the pelvis. Its lower end enters the vagina and is called the cervix, and its upper ends attach to the Fallopian tubes. This upper part of the uterus is called the body of the uterus. Cancer arising in the lower part of the uterus, the cervix, is known as cervical cancer, while cancer arising in the body of the uterus is known as uterine cancer or endometrial cancer, the reasons for which I shall shortly explain. The distinction between these two types of cancer – cervical and uterine – is essential to an understanding of this subject.

Finally, another important aspect of definition. The wall of the uterus is made up of muscle. Areas of this muscle can sometimes undergo abnormal growth, forming small round knots of muscular tissue known as fibroids. Doctors sometimes refer to these fibroids as tumours, which, although technically correct, can often lead to total misunderstanding on the part of the patient, as fibroids are non-cancerous.

What causes cervical cancer?

The exact cause of cervical cancer is not known although a number of predisposing factors are recognized. However, I would like to state most emphatically that these predisposing factors are the result of statistical surveys, and one of the main problems with these surveys is that they tend to overlook the individual and the personal nature of a disease or problem. It is disconcerting to see oneself categorized as being a certain 'sort of person' because one is suffering from a particular disease. This is particularly the case when talking about the predisposing factors of cervical cancer. There are many high-risk groups for this disease but this does not mean to say that if you have cervical cancer you necessarily belong to any of these groups.

It is currently believed that cervical cancer is caused by a virus which may possibly be transmitted by sexual intercourse.

It is also said that cervical cancer is more common in groups of women who have had more than one partner, the incidence apparently increasing with the more partners that the woman has had. However, this bland statistic takes no account of the numbers of partners that the males may have had (there seem to be no statistics available for this angle of the problem), all of which gives a somewhat biased and one-sided interpretation of the facts.

What causes uterine cancer?

Uterine cancer, or cancer of the body of the uterus, is often referred to as endometrial cancer. The endometrium is a particular part of the body of the uterus, the inner lining (within which the fertilized ovum embeds itself after conception and develops into the foetus). It is here that uterine cancer occurs.

One of the important differences between uterine cancer and cancer of the cervix is that uterine cancer seems to arise later in life, often after the menopause and in women who have had no children. Statistically, obese women and those who have diabetes are more likely to develop the disease.

The exact way in which uterine cancer develops is not known, though it is thought that hormonal imbalance may play a part.

What happens if cancer of the cervix is discovered during pregnancy?

This diagnosis always poses a particularly difficult problem. If the cancer is at a very early stage then as long as it is closely observed throughout the pregnancy treatment can wait until after delivery. Where the cancer is more advanced, account must be taken of the stage of the pregnancy and, of course, how the woman feels about the pregnancy and the way in which it affects the cancer of her cervix.

The principles of treatment are the same as for those cases with cancer of the cervix not occurring in pregnancy. If the cancer is diagnosed later in pregnancy there is always the possibility of performing a Caesarean section to deliver a healthy baby before treatement is started.

The problem of cervical cancer being discovered in pregnancy is yet another important reminder of how vital it is for all women to have routine cervical screening.

Can uterine or cervical cancer be detected before symptoms develop?

Uterine cancer is almost impossible to detect in the absence of symptoms. The complete reverse is true of cancer of the cervix. This cancer, above all others, is eminently detectable by routine screening procedures. Figures show that since routine cervical screening for cancer became standard practice the number of cases of advanced cervical cancer has decreased dramatically. Although the disease undoubtedly still occurs, as a result of these procedures it can be picked up in the earliest stages of its development when treatment can normally be completely curative.

The message is very simple. *Cervical screening for cancer is an essential investigation that should routinely be done on all women.*

Ideally every woman should have a cervical smear done once a year. Ask your own doctor what his policy on the matter is, and follow his advice.

Having a cervical smear test is a painless procedure and is easily arranged. You can have it done either at your Family Planning Clinic or at your own doctor's surgery. The procedure is very simple. Following an internal examination, the doctor will pass a spatula (which looks rather like a lollipop stick) over the opening of the cervix. The superficial cells of the cervix are thus transferred to the spatula which in turn is rubbed on a glass slide. The slide is then taken to the pathology laboratory where the cervical cells on it are examined. By looking at the cells under the microscope the cytologist who does this examination will be able to decide whether they are normal, premalignant or malignant. I cannot over-emphasize that this simple test, which is painless and takes only five minutes, can be a real life-saver.

What are the symptoms of uterine cancer?

Like so many symptoms of cancer generally, the initial symptoms of cancer of the uterus can appear to be innocuous. They are, therefore, often ignored for long periods, the assumption being that they will just go away. The causes of these symptoms will often be found to be due to benign problems such as cervical erosions, uterine fibroids or disturbed menstrual bleeding. However, it is important to ensure that a diagnosis of cancer is excluded before assuming that the problem is due to one of these causes.

Another mistake is to assume that, having once had a diagnosis made of a benign problem, recent symptoms are due to this former problem. In short, then, if you have symptoms – *any* symptoms – never put them down to a previous problem; go and have them fully checked out.

Uterine cancer tends to arise in women over the age of 40 and particularly after the menopause. Any bloody vaginal discharge after the menopause should be reported to your doctor immediately. In women who have not yet reached the menopause the signs can be irregular or unusual bleeding. This can take the form of bleeding after intercourse, bleeding between periods, or heavier than normal bleeding at period time. Unpleasant vaginal discharges can sometimes also be an early symptom. If you have any of these signs or symptoms, therefore, do not hesitate to seek the advice of your doctor. There will normally be a perfectly innocent explanation such as dysfunctional uterine bleeding, fibroids or a cervical erosion but the diagnosis of cancer must not be overlooked or excluded.

What are the symptoms of cervical cancer?

This cancer tends to occur in a younger age group than uterine cancer.

The symptoms are similar to those of uterine cancer, however, in that there is abnormal bleeding in the form of bleeding between periods, bleeding after intercourse or particularly heavy periods. An offensive and watery vaginal discharge is also sometimes experienced.

If you have one or more of these symptoms, seek medical advice.

What sort of tests will I have to have?

Although your GP or the doctor at the Family Planning Clinic will examine your womb you will almost certainly be asked to attend the gynaecological department at your local hospital.

Your consultant gynaecologist will probably advise that you come into hospital for a 24-hour period for an investigation commonly known as a 'D and C' (dilatation and curettage), which involves the following. You will be taken to theatre and given a general anaesthetic. Then the small opening in the neck of your cervix will be gently dilated and through this dilated opening a curette will be passed. The curette will gather sample tissue from the endometrium (lining of the uterus) which is sent to the pathology laboratory for examination for malignant cells.

While you are under the general anaesthetic your consultant will also perform a manual examination of your uterus to see whether or not a tumour can be felt.

You will normally be allowed to leave hospital the day following this procedure, and even sometimes on the same day. For the next few days you may notice a slight and variable amount of vaginal discharge and bleeding.

If cervical cancer is suspected your consultant gynaecologist will normally be able to assess whether or not this problem is present during examination, in the out-patients department. Cancer of the cervix, as opposed to pre-cervical cancer, can normally be seen by direct visual inspection with the use of a magnifying instrument known as a colposcope. The consultant will then probably do a further cervical smear together with what is known as a punch biopsy. This is a painless procedure but is important for it will reveal the extent to which the cancerous cells have spread.

If the investigations show that you have cancer of the uterus or cervix your consultant may order some further investigations to establish how far the cancer has progressed. You may, for example, have an ultrasound scan of the uterus to establish the size of the cancer. A CAT scan of the abdomen and pelvis may be done to establish whether or not the cancer has spread outside the confines of the uterus, and an intravenous pyelogram (p.34) is sometimes performed to establish whether or not the ureters, which carry the urine from the kidneys to the bladder and pass very close to the uterus, are involved.

How is uterine cancer treated?

This will depend to a large extent on how far the cancer has spread. The extent of the cancerous spread can be staged; the particular stages being assessed by the investigation described earlier. In Stage 1 of the disease the cancer is confined within the uterus. Stage 2 denotes a spread to the cervix. Stage 3 is where the cancer has spread beyond the uterus and Stage 4 occurs when the cancer has spread to involve adjacent structures such as the bladder.

If the cancer is confined to the uterus (Stages 1 or 2) then surgery is advised. This involves a hysterectomy (removal of the uterus), together with the removal of the Fallopian tubes and the ovaries, known as bilateral oophorectomy. Cancers that have spread beyond the uterus are normally treated by radiotherapy alone.

External or internal radiotherapy (see pp.45-47) may also be given before or after the operation.

How is cancer of the cervix treated?

Preliminary investigations will already have revealed how far the cancer has spread. At its earliest stage, Stage 1, the cancer has not spread beyond the confines of the cervix. The outlook for successful treatment at this stage is extremely good.

There are two surgical approaches that can be made. One possibility is a cone biopsy. This involves removing only that part of the cervical tissue that is affected by malignant change. A hysterectomy is not done but regular check-ups are essential to make sure that the cancer does not reappear.

An alternative treatment at this early stage is hysterectomy. This procedure will ensure an almost 100 per cent cure and the problem is eradicated for ever. Some surgeons will combine hysterectomy with the removal of the ovaries; others perform a hysterectomy, leaving the ovaries. In pre-menopausal women whose ovaries are removed, hormone replacement therapy substitutes for the loss of the natural ovarian hormones.

An alternative for early cervical cancer is radiotherapy. Treatment for Stage 2 cervical cancer (additional spread to the vagina) depends upon the way in which the cancer has spread in the cervix. If it has spread to involve just a small part of the upper part of the vagina then hysterectomy together with radiotherapy is normally advised.

Stage 3 (involving further spread to the vagina as well as local spread to other pelvic structures) and Stage 4 (metastatic spread, together with spread to the bladder or bowel) are normally treated by radiotherapy alone. Sometimes it is given by placing a radioactive compound within the cervix, known as intracavitary treatment. This may also be combined with external radiation therapy.

Intracavitary radiotherapy is normally given on two separate occasions, the radioactive source being placed in the cervix for about 24 hours.

To avoid excessive radiation to the surrounding structures such as the bladder and the bowel these treatments are normally given with an interval of two to three weeks between them.

What sort of problems can occur after a hysterectomy?

Problems after a hysterectomy can be both physical and psychological.

As with any operation, a certain amount of time has to be given over to allowing the tissues to heal. A hysterectomy can be misleading because outwardly there may be little in the way of a sign that you have had an operation, apart from a very small scar on your lower abdomen. This belies the fact that the tissues of your pelvic floor will have been weakened by the operation. Your physiotherapist will encourage you to do pelvic floor exercises to strengthen your pelvic muscles, but physical activity such as lifting heavy weights (e.g. moving furniture; lifting heavy piles of washing; carrying heavy bags of shopping) should not be undertaken for six weeks following the operation.

Sexual activity is physically not restricted by hysterectomy though even three months after the operation slight discomfort may be felt. It is normally advised that intercourse should not take place for at least six weeks after the operation and then only gently at first.

If you are in any doubt as to do's and don'ts ask your consultant's advice at your first outpatient's appointment.

The psychological problems of hysterectomy are not discussed nearly as openly as they should be. If they were, they would soon cease to exist. What can be stated quite categorically is that there is no physical reason for any loss of libido or restriction of normal sexual activity following a hysterectomy. In fact, many women describe improved sexual relations and a sense of relief after the operation, not only because their problem has been successfully treated but because they also feel physically better.

When discussing psychological problems associated with hysterectomy the partner should not be forgotten. His silent fears may include the mistaken belief that sexual intercourse can no longer occur. He may feel that the hysterectomy could have a serious effect on the physical relationship that he has with his partner. Some men may even worry that they can catch cancer from their partners. All these fears are unfounded but, to some men, are very real.

Again, I must emphasize that both partners should ask the consultant gynaecologist what the woman should do following her hysterectomy, in terms of normal daily activities and lifestyle as well as how and when normal sexual relationships can be commenced.

If problems occur with either partner these should be discussed with your GP and, if necessary, with a psychologist with training in this area.

What is cancer of the stomach?

Cancer of the stomach is the most common cancer of the upper digestive tract, although the term 'stomach cancer' is in fact a blanket term that describes three types of cancer that can develop in this area. The first of these looks very much like an ulcer arising in the inner wall of the stomach (not to be confused with a benign stomach ulcer, see below). The second, known as a polypoid tumour, grows from the inner lining of the stomach wall into the stomach cavity. The third is known as the 'leather bottle' stomach cancer, and occurs when the whole of the stomach wall is infiltrated by cancerous tissue.

What causes cancer of the stomach?

The definitive cause of stomach cancer is not known. There are, though, a number of factors suggesting that the probable cause or causes are environmental and dietary.

In Japan, cancer of the stomach is a common disease. Consequently, the Japanese have been extensively investigated and a number of factors in the diet of Japanese gastric cancer sufferers have been mooted as possible causes. It has been shown, for example, that certain forms of rice can be contaminated with asbestos, though this type of contamination is not considered to be a major problem worldwide. Suspicion has also fallen upon nitrates, commonly used as fertilizers both in Japan and elsewhere in the world, and on high levels of lead and zinc in the water supply. Examination of the socio-economic grouping of these cancer sufferers revealed that the vast majority are in the lowest socio-economic grouping. Such a grouping necessarily suggests a poor diet but whether this is due to lack of certain dietary constituents or a high intake of poor-quality food is not known.

Genetic factors have also been implanted in the evidence of stomach cancer. These have been well-documented, albeit rare, studies of families and twins with a high incidence of stomach cancer. Rather broader genetic evidence comes from the fact that people of blood group A are known to be more prone to developing gastric cancer than the remainder of the population (blood group A is, necessarily, an inherited characteristic). A rare form of anaemia, called pernicious anaemia, caused by lack of vitamin B12, can also be statistically associated with stomach cancer but whether this is a genetic or an environmental feature still remains a mystery.

As to predisposing diseases of the stomach, there are conflicting pieces of evidence. It has been suggested that stomach cancer, in rare instances, can arise in or around a chronic gastric ulcer, which in turn is believed to be caused by high acid content of the stomach. Conversely, in conditions of undersecretion of acid in the stomach – a condition known as achlorhydria – gastric cancer is also said to show an increased incidence. So, gastric cancer would appear to be caused by environmental factors, and specifically a dietary factor which would appear to cause its effects in an individual who has both a genetic predisposition to the disease and an abnormal secretion of acid in his stomach.

What are the symptoms of stomach cancer?

Although there are symptoms of cancer of the stomach, these are non-specific, being similar to those of a gastric ulcer and general upsets of the upper gastro-intestinal tract. Such symptoms, nebulous though they may be, only serve to emphasize how important it is that they be thoroughly investigated by your GP.

For example, you may notice that you are losing weight without trying to do so. People may say that you are looking paler than usual. You may have felt off-colour for a month or two. Combined with these vague symptoms you may notice that you experience a dull ache in the upper part of your abdomen. You may also find that you have a feeling of fullness in your stomach, that somehow you are unable to digest your food as easily as you used to. Chronic indigestion may become a problem. Although you may ignore some of these signs and symptoms the one symptom that must never be ignored is the vomiting up of blood, even if it is only a trace. The most common cause of vomiting blood is in fact normally not cancer but a benign ulcer, either gastric or duodenal, but this symptom must not be dismissed and should be reported to your doctor immediately.

What tests will I have to have?

The first test you have will probably be a barium meal. Your GP will normally arrange this investigation directly with the radiology department at the hospital. After the appointment is made you should receive a list of instructions, the most important of which will be to ask you not to eat or drink anything for a variable amount of time before the test. Once at the radiology department you will be asked to drink what looks like a simple glass of milk but which is in fact a radio-opaque liquid called barium. As the barium passes down into your stomach the radiologist, who will be conducting the examination, will be able to observe its passage into and through your stomach and duodenum. The lining of your stomach wall will be outlined by the barium, which is seen on the X-ray as a dense white area. By looking at this carefully, the radiologist will observe any suspicious-looking areas and, by considering their size and position can, in a large percentage of cases, diagnose their nature.

The whole test takes, on average, an hour, during which, in order for the whole of the lining of the stomach to be examined, it will be necessary to move you into a series of different positions. The procedure is painless, however, and causes no discomfort (though some people do not like the taste of the barium).

Following this examination, a closer inspection of a suspicious area is sometimes required. Under such circumstances a gastroscopy may be recommended. This test is usually done on an outpatient basis though, because a mild sedative is normally used, time must be allowed, afterwards, for recovery. It is best, therefore, to ensure that someone is waiting to take you home after the test has finished.

Gastroscopy involves passing a gastroscope (a fibre-optic tube) down the gullet and into the stomach. The light properties of the fibre-optical system allow the doctor to see down the gastroscope and into and around the various internal aspects of your stomach. In this way the inner lining of the stomach can be directly visualized.

As with the barium meal you will be asked not to eat or drink for a variable amount of time before the examination in order to clear the stomach of all residual contents. You may feel some discomfort as the gastroscope is passed down your gullet, but a sedative will be given to relieve this. In addition, a local anaesthetic will be sprayed on the back of your tongue to deaden your gag reflex and allow for easier passage of the gastroscope.

Even by direct visualization, your doctor may not be able to decide whether or not the ulcer he is looking at is cancerous or benign, but one of the advantages of the gastroscopy is that he can use the fibre-optiscope to take a small biopsy which can later be examined in the laboratory for the presence or absence of cancerous tissue.

How is cancer of the stomach treated?

If at all possible, the cancerous stomach is removed by surgery. This procedure is known as gastrectomy. Surgery is the mainstay of treatment though in a certain number of cases, the condition may be too advanced for surgery to be deemed successful.

Gastrectomy is a major procedure which, inevitably, is carried out on people who are not in the best state of health, all of which can add to the long-term problems associated with the operation. In addition to surgery, chemotherapy may be given. The drug most commonly used is

5-Flurouracil which can be taken orally or intravenously.

In the immediate post-operative period, blood loss from the operation, as well as the anaemia caused by the gastric cancer, may necessitate a blood transfusion. Other more general problems posed by post-operative gastrectomy are those of breathing and diet. As far as breathing is concerned, immediately after the operation, your physiotherapist will instruct you in deep breathing techniques. She will also encourage early mobilization – even if this only means sitting out of bed – because this will allow the diaphragm to drop more easily, which consequently allows for easier lung expansion.

In the immediate post-operative period it is important to build up your strength. This may mean parenteral feeding: giving carbohydrates, proteins and fat by way of an intravenous infusion. In the immediate post-operative period food by mouth will not be allowed.

In the longer term, problems with diet may occur because of the absence of the stomach. Biologically the stomach has a vital role to play in supplying the body with a vitamin called B12. This vitamin is essential for the normal production of red blood cells and without it a form of anaemia called pernicious anaemia develops. Following a gastrectomy, therefore, B12 supplements have to be given as intramuscular injections on a maintenance basis.

In addition, for digestive comfort it will be recommended that you take smaller, but more frequent, meals.

What is skin cancer?

This is a blanket term describing several cancers of the skin. Two common forms are malignant melanoma and rodent ulcer.

What is a malignant melanoma?

As with other cancers, early recognition is important because the sooner the condition is diagnosed and treated the better are the chances of recovery. Although a malignant melanoma appears as a rather small, innocuous area on the skin, it is a rapidly spreading form of cancer, which extends with relative ease through the lymphatic system to sites such as the liver and brain. This cancer can arise in existing, benign skin moles that you may have had all your life.

What are the symptoms of malignant melanoma?

A malignant melanoma can arise in either a pre-existing mole or freckle or on an area of previously unblemished skin. Its size is normally small, no larger than an average-sized mole or freckle. Slight changes in existing moles can often go unnoticed. The signs to look out for are as follows.

There may be a change in colour. It is a common misconception that a melanoma changes from a light colour to a dark colour. This is the case in certain circumstances but some melanomas, as they develop, become lighter in colour. Altenatively, parts of the melanoma may show uneven, mottled colouring – mixtures of red, grey, blue or even white areas. The essential thing to look for is any change in colour.

Look also at the border of the suspicious area. Normally moles have a smooth raised border. A change from a smooth border to an irregular border is suspicious. A change in the shape of a mole or blemish may also indicate that a malignant melanoma is developing within it. A change of shape may include a change in size as well as a change in the regularity of the surface of the mole. The surface may become irregular with small, uneven bumps on it.

Other very important warning signs that should never be ignored are spontaneous ulceration or bleeding of a previously normal mole. Before any of these rather more obvious signs become apparent, the developing melanoma may also give the sensation of itching or irritation.

Again, this must not be ignored. Any of the symptoms described above can be due to a harmless skin condition. Nevertheless, if you notice any of these features developing in either a mole or an area of previously unblemished skin, take the problem to your doctor.

What causes a malignant melanoma?

There are a number of predisposing factors which are thought to influence the development of a malignant melanoma. The cells in the skin which become malignant are called melanocytes. These are the cells that are normally responsible for skin pigmentation and it is according to their numbers and activity that the colour of the skin is determined.

The cause of malignant melanoma is believed, in part, to be related to the effect of bright light on fair skin. It has been shown that in fair-skinned populations, such as those found in Australia, exposure to bright light can markedly increase the overall incidence of the occurrence of malignant melonomas.

Surveys carried out in Israel have shown a definite correlation between exposure to sunlight in fair-skinned individuals and the development of malignant melanomas.

Melanomas are less commonly seen in dark-skinned races. When they *are* seen in these races, the sites of development of the melanomas are on lighter areas of the skin such as the sole of the foot. However, it is probably too simplistic to speculate from all this that direct sunlight, in itself, causes cancerous changes in the melanocytic cells.

It is believed that melanomas which develop in pre-existing moles originate within specific skin cells known as junctional naevi cells. These are particularly unstable cells and it is known that a stimulus such as excessive sunlight can change these junctional cells into malignant cells.

Can malignant melanoma be prevented and how is it treated?

Although direct prevention itself is not possible, it is important to emphasize that there are certain people who are more at risk than others.

The highest risk group are fair-skinned individuals working and living for lengthy periods in countries where sunlight is both bright and prolonged. This includes people who have emigrated to countries where these conditions exist. The world's workforce is increasingly more mobile and many fair-skinned individuals can find themselves spending a considerable part of their working life in hot and sunny climates. It is important that such people in particular do not delay in getting medical help if they recognize any of symptoms that I have mentioned.

Malignant melanoma is treated as follows. When you go to your GP, he may be able to reassure you instantly that your condition is benign. If he is unsure, he will refer you to a dermatologist (a specialist who specializes in skin conditions). The dermatologist will be in a position to state, by looking at the suspicious skin lesion, whether or not it is malignant. However, even if he feels that it is not malignant, he will normally advise that it be treated as such as a safety precaution. This means surgically removing the mole, together with a margin of the surrounding skin. Sometimes a skin graft will have to be placed over the area of skin deficit that remains. If, on examination, the mole is found to be malignant, the local lymph nodes may also be surgically removed.

You will recall that a common way in which malignant melanoma spreads is by the lymphatic system. Such lymphatics flow to lymph nodes and some surgeons will advise that these draining lymph nodes should also be excised. This operation is known as block dissection of the lymph nodes.

What is a rodent ulcer?

A rodent ulcer, also known as a basal cell carcinoma, is, like malignant melanoma, a form of skin cancer. Although these lesions are commonly referred to as rodent ulcers they are cancerous. That said, they are a very innocuous form of cancer and are eminently treatable and curable.

Rodent ulcers usually appear on areas of the body that are exposed to sunlight, and most commonly on the face. A rodent ulcer may often easily go unnoticed because in its initial stage it appears as just a small lump within the skin. There is no marked colour change of this lump or in the skin surrounding the lump. But, as the lesion grows, a small depression develops in its centre. Sometimes, too, the skin over the rodent ulcer can ulcerate and bleed spontaneously.

How is a rodent ulcer treated?

As mentioned earlier, this is a form of cancer that can truly be said to be curable, and the various treatments for the condition are extremely effective. The type of treatment will depend upon the site of the rodent ulcer. One method is surgical removal, in which the ulcer is simply cut out under local anaesthetic. In some cases, a small skin graft may have to be inserted to replace any skin deficit.

Another method of treating rodent ulcers is by external radiotherapy (see p.45). Following this type of therapy, the treated skin may sometimes look somewhat paler than the surrounding skin, but such blemishes can easily be covered up with cosmetics.

Some dermatologists may also advise cryotherapy, where a low temperature probe is placed on the ulcer, the cancerous cells being destroyed by the very low temperature.

What is cancer of the prostate?

The prostate gland is found in men at the base of the bladder. It surrounds part of the urethra (the passage that allows urine to drain from the bladder). Enlargement of this gland is a condition that can give rise to urinary difficulties. However, such enlargement is not necessarily due to cancer. In the majority of cases it is caused by a condition known as benign prostatic hyperplasia – a uniform enlargement of the gland which is a very common condition found in men over the age of 60.

Prostatic cancer can either develop of its own accord or arise in a gland that is already showing signs of enlargement. The symptoms of this type of cancer are very difficult to distinguish from those of benign prostatic hyperplasia (both referred to as prostatism).

Whatever the cause of these symptoms, therefore, they must be thoroughly investigated. Not only is there a danger with prostatic cancer of the cancer spreading and growing to involve surrounding structures but, both in the case of prostatic cancer and benign prostatic hyperplasia, urinary retention can occur.

What are the symptoms of prostatism?

The following are warning signs of enlargement of the prostate gland from whatever cause. The earliest sign is known as frequency, which describes the need to pass urine frequently. Normally, frequency begins at night, the patient having to get up two or three times to pass urine. Then, after a variable amount of time, it begins to become part of the daily routine. Superimposed upon this daily frequency is another symptom known as urgency. This describes an intense need to urinate, though, when the need is met, little urine is actually passed.

As these stages progress, other symptoms arise, such as terminal dribbling (a prolongation of urination after emptying the bladder). There may also be difficulty in starting to urinate, with straining only making the problem worse. Once urination does begin, the stream is variable and often intermittent. Urination can also become painful and on occasions blood may be passed in the urine.

If you have any of these signs or symptoms, report them to your doctor. If you do not, you may go on to develop what is known as acute retention of urine. This occurs when the urethra becomes completely blocked and urine builds up in the bladder. The patient is unable to pass urine and, at the same time, the bladder swelling causes acute lower abdominal discomfort. Acute retention of urine is an emergency and will mean having to go to hospital, where a catheter will be passed into the bladder to release the retained urine. Hopefully, when you seek medical assistance for your prostatic problems it will not be as a result of an acute urinary retention.

The initial examination that your doctor will make will be a rectal examination. The prostate gland lies just in front of the anal canal and its shape can be felt through the wall of the anal canal. The shape can often be a vital clue to the underlying nature of the prostatic enlargement. A smooth enlarged gland is invariably benign prostatic hyperplasia, whereas a gland that is unevenly enlarged may be cancerous.

Though, having said this, often when a seemingly benign enlarged prostate gland has been removed and is examined in the pathology laboratory it is sometimes shown to be cancerous

Cancer often develops in a prostate gland that is showing signs of benign prostatic hyperplasia but what actually sparks off this change is not known.

How are these prostatic problems investigated?

Even if your GP does not suspect prostatic cancer he will probably refer you to a urologist (consultant surgeon who specializes in urinary problems). Like your own doctor, he will examine your prostate gland. At the same time he will take what is known as a 'needle biopsy' of the gland itself. This is a painless procedure and is done in the outpatients department. It involves a needle being passed into the prostate gland and a small specimen of tissue being taken from it and later examined in the pathology laboratory for any evidence of malignant cells. A blood test will also be ordered to look for a specific chemical known as acid phosphatase which is produced by cancerous growth in the prostate gland. If the level of acid phosphatase is raised and the biopsy specimen demonstrates that there is evidence of cancer of the prostate you will probably have a bone scan. This is a specialized survey of your bones to look for any evidence of spread of the prostatic cancer. You will also have an intravenous pyelogram (see p.34) – a series of X-rays that will look at the functioning of your urinary system.

How is prostatic cancer treated?

In many instances, prostatic cancer is diagnosed following a routine operation for removal of an enlarged prostate (prostatectomy).

In some cases, therefore, it is unintentionally, though correctly, surgically removed, thus solving the problem (assuming that there has been no spread of the prostatic cancer elsewhere).

Pre-diagnosed prostatic cancer can be treated either by surgery or radiotherapy or a combination of the two. As far as surgery is concerned there are two basic prostatectomy operations. The first is a lower abdominal operation in which the surgeon will remove the prostate gland from the pelvis. The second is a procedure whereby a diathermy probe is passed through the urethra and the prostate gland is removed internally without the need for abdominal surgery. The technique used will depend upon the size and nature of the prostatic enlargement.

One of the problems associated with surgical prostatectomy is sexual impotence. There is also a possibility that some patients may be left with a degree of post-operative urinary incontinence.

Sometimes radiotherapy is used as a method of treatment, with or without surgery. External radiotherapy (see p.45) can be given but many radiotherapists believe that the most efficient way of irradiating the cancer in the prostate gland is by inserting implants of radioactive material into the gland.

One of the advantages of radiotherapy over surgery is that sexual impotence is much less of a problem as are the problems of urinary incontinence.

On pp.8-22, when discussing the causes of cancer, I mentioned that certain cancers were hormone-dependent. This feature is especially true of prostatic cancer in that the growth of this cancer is helped by the male hormone testosterone, which is produced in the testicles. Reduction of testosterone levels in the bloodstream can be achieved by giving the female hormone oestrogen, taken in tablet form. This method of reducing the growth of prostatic cancer is useful when treating the spread of prostatic cancer, especially when it extends into the bones where it can be particularly painful. The only drawback to the use of oestrogens is that, in some cases, they can hasten the onset of arteriosclerosis of the blood vessels with consequent cardiovascular problems. These potential side-effects have to be balanced, therefore, against the likely benefits. Because of these side-effects, regular cardiovascular check-ups will be recommended for patients on oestrogen treatment.

Does the phrase 'brain tumour' necessarily mean cancer of the brain?

The term brain tumour refers to abnormal growth of tissue in the brain, but tissue that demonstrates abnormal growth is not necessarily cancerous. The human brain is an extremely complex structure made up of several different types of nerve tissue, each tissue being capable of undergoing abnormal growth. Consequently the list of both cancerous and non-cancerous growths in the brain is long. Tumours of the brain, by which I mean both cancerous and non-cancerous growths, can be divided into two main groups: areas of cancerous growth which have spread from cancers elsewhere in the body and benign or cancerous growths that arise from the brain substance itself. Areas of growth which have spread from cancer elsewhere are referred to as 'secondary deposits', also known as metastases. These secondary islands of cancerous cells are carried from their primary site to the brain in the bloodstream. They are normally late manifestations of cancer and evidence of advanced growth of a primary tumour. Occasionally, their detection may be the first evidence of a cancer somewhere else within the body.

Of the tumours arising from the brain itself, some are cancerous and others benign. To take the non-cancerous brain tumours first: one of the most common of these is known as meningioma. This tumour does not arise from the brain itself but from the meninges (linings of the brain). Another form of non-malignant brain tumour is the acoustic neuroma. This benign tumour grows from the auditory nerve which conveys the sensation of hearing. A third group of non-malignant brain tumours are those from the pituitary gland, which lies under the brain and is the 'headquarters' of the body's hormonal system. Growths can occur in various parts of the pituitary gland and, although non-cancerous, may cause a variety of bodily effects due either to over-production or underproduction of various hormones.

Let us turn now to the true cancerous growths of the brain. These are rare and this fact should be remembered if you are worried that you may be experiencing the symptoms of a brain tumour. Needless to say, however, any such symptoms should never be ignored.

There are a number of different primary cancerous brain tumours, collectively referred to as the neurogliomas. There is no hard evidence as to the exact cause of these tumours though, in some, suspicion has fallen on a viral agent which may be responsible for initiating the cancer. Evidence for this has largely been accumulated from examination of these tumours in cell culture where viral particles have been identified.

What are the symptoms of brain tumours?

Like so many other cancers the symptoms of brain tumours are often non-specific. As I have emphasized, cancerous tumours arising in the brain itself are particularly rare. Having said that, symptoms of brain tumours should not be ignored even though the statistical likelihood of having a brain tumour diagnosed is slight. Tumours produce many symptoms, which will vary according to the site of the tumour in the brain. For instance, you will recall that I mentioned the pituitary gland and the way in which non-cancerous tumours of this gland can cause hormonal effects. An example of overproduction of one of the hormones from this gland, the growth hormone, may cause an increase in size of some of the bones of the body resulting in a condition known as acromegaly.

Another form of pituitary tumour secretes a hormone called ACTH

(Adrenocorticotrophic hormone) which, in turn, stimulates the adrenal gland causing it to overproduce steroid hormones resulting in a disease known as Cushing's syndrome. These two examples demonstrate the diversity of the effects and symptoms of certain brain tumours.

The expansion of pituitary tumours can also cause loss of vision due to their growth and subsequent pressure on the optic nerve. This is an example of a tumour having what is known as a 'local' effect, disrupting the function of a structure in its immediate vicinity. Similarly, an acoustic neuroma, another non-cancerous benign tumour, can cause deafness by growing into the auditory nerve.

A third type of non-cancerous brain tumour, a meningioma, can impinge upon nerves that work the eye muscles. This may result in double vision, a further example of a local effect. All this serves to demonstrate the importance of recognizing the diverse symptoms that each type of brain tumour can give.

Let us turn now to the true cancerous tumours of the brain: the neurogliomas and the metastatic tumours. Such tumours grow at different rates but their growth may eventually cause raised intracranial pressure. This occurs because the brain is essentially a soft structure surrounded by a rigid protective coating, the skull. Any increase in the volume of the structures within the skull will precipitate a variety of symptoms. Initially there will be headaches. Headaches due to brain tumours are often worse in the morning rather than later in the day, though this is by no means always the case. Sensations of nausea and sickness may also develop and eventually unexplained vomiting may occur. In addition, the optic nerves may become compressed and swollen, a condition known as papilloedema. This is noticed as varying degrees of loss of vision.

One important general effect of raised intracranial pressure that should be noted is an epileptic attack or seizure (though it is very important to stress that the vast majority of epileptic attacks have nothing to do with brain tumours).

Due to the raised intracranial pressure, nerves to the eye muscles may become compressed, also resulting in double vision.

There are also some rather more nebulous signs and symptoms which may be due to brain tumours. Examples of these are changes in personality (signs that may be mistaken for senile dementia), and difficulty in recognizing objects and expressing ideas.

It is important to remember that such symptoms can be due to many diseases both in the brain and in the rest of the body and that just because you have these symptoms does not mean that you have a brain tumour. However, do not ignore these symptoms, especially if you notice them in a relative.

How are brain tumours investigated?

If your GP suspects that you might have a brain tumour he will send you to a specialist called a neurologist. Following a full examination the neurologist will order a series of tests.

Over recent years the diagnosis of brain tumours has undergone a revolution. In the past it used to be a protracted and sometimes painful series of investigations, and it is because of this that many myths still remain about discomfort experienced in neurological tests. However, with the advent of computerized tomography (also known as CT scanning or CAT scan) everything has changed. Computerized tomography is a sophisticated computerized X-ray machine that works on the same basic principle as the ordinary X-ray but is able to give much more detailed and clearer pictures.

The machine is itself large, and some patients are put off by its size, but the procedure, although quite time consuming, is entirely painless.

If there has been any hint of an epileptic attack you will also undergo what is known as an EEG (electroencephalogram). This entails positioning a number of small electrodes over your skull to pick up the electrical activity of your brain. Epilepsy is abnormal electrical activity in a part of your brain which can be detected by the EEG machine.

Sometimes, in order to accurately locate the position of a brain tumour, a further investigation called an angiogram will be done. This involves injecting a dye into the arterial system which, under X-ray screening, will demonstrate the particular nature of the blood supply to the tumour. This can be of great help to the surgeon in planning his operative approach.

How are brain tumours treated?

Many patients with brain tumours will undergo surgery. The surgery may be curative, or may be done to relieve raised intracranial pressure or the symptoms caused by the tumour. Additionally, surgery may also allow a biopsy of the tumour tissue in order to establish an accurate diagnosis and to plan further treatment.

There are a number of different surgical procedures to tackle the many different sorts of brain tumour. Although I cannot go into specific details about them all here, there are some points which I should like to mention about the general principles surrounding neurosurgery that are of interest from a patient's point of view.

With benign cranial tumours, including tumours of the pituitary gland, acoustic neuromas and meningiomas, the success rate in the removal of these tumours is high. Much depends upon the stage at which they were detected and the reversibility of their compressive effects.

In the case of removal of acoustic neuromas, a variable amount of hearing loss may have to be accepted, while long-term hormonal replacement is normally required after removal of the pituitary gland. Removal of meningiomas, on the other hand, has no long-term lasting effects.

However the cancerous tumours pose a more difficult problem. This is because, unlike the benign brain tumours, they are not localized but tend to spread and merge into the surrounding healthy brain tissue.

In some instances they are so close to vitally important areas of the brain that it is sometimes too dangerous to attempt their removal.

With the advancement of microsurgical techniques, however, such tumours can now more easily be tackled. If the tumour has caused excessive swelling in the brain it is often necessary to reduce this swelling before the operation takes place. This is done by using a steroid drug called dexamethasone, which can either be injected or taken by mouth.

Preparations for neurosurgery are no different to other forms of surgery, the main difference being that, in most instances, it is necessary to completely shave the head.

During the post-operative period there will often be headaches. These are always treated with pain-killing drugs and will never be long-lasting.

Radiotherapy may be used independently or combined with surgery. With some pituitary gland tumours, radiotherapy can treat the problem though normally these tumours are treated by surgery.

What is leukaemia?

Leukaemia is a cancer of certain white blood cells. It is not one specific disease, but, rather, a blanket term that covers several different diseases. Probably the easiest way to understand leukaemia is to look at the way in which white blood cells are normally formed and then to see how this normal process of blood cell formation can become cancerous.

Blood cells can be divided into red cells, white cells and platelets. Each type of cell has a different function. Red blood cells (erythrocytes) aid the body's metabolism by carrying oxygen to the tissues and carbon dioxide from them; white blood cells are of two varieties, lymphocytes and leucocytes, and defend the body from both infection and cancerous growth; platelets are an important part of the blood's clotting mechanism, responsible for stopping bleeding. Each of these three varieties of cells is produced in the bone marrow, a specialized tissue found in the central areas of bones.

All these cells develop from primitive cells known as stem cells. They have a rapid turnover, the lifespan of each cell normally being only weeks or a few months, at most. This inevitably means that they are being produced at an enormous rate. It is not hard to imagine how these bone marrow cells can, if the control of this process is disturbed, move from a smooth production of normal cells into a phase of overproduction which may then merge into a cancerous change termed leukaemia (cancer of the white cells). The problem with these leukaemic cells is not simply that they are overproduced but also that they are functionally immature. In other words, they are unable to carry out their normal functions. As we shall see, this is a major cause of the symptoms of leukaemia.

Are there different forms of leukaemia?

There are various forms of leukaemia and they can be divided into two main groups: acute and chronic. These terms refer to both the speed of onset and, to a certain extent, the outcome. There are two forms of chronic leukaemia: chronic myeloid leukaemia and chronic lymphatic leukaemia. There are also two forms of acute leukaemia: acute myeloid leukaemia and acute lymphatic leukaemia.

Before proceeding with these, however, I would like to discuss two further diseases: multiple myeloma and Hodgkin's disease. Although neither of these is a leukaemia both are related to leukaemias in that their cellular proliferation and cancerous changes are closely related to the family of cells that are concerned in the leukaemic process.

Let us first look at multiple myeloma. When describing the white cells I mentioned that their function was one of defence. Amongst the white cells is a group of cells referred to as plasma cells.

These plasma cells are found in bone marrow and, like white cells, are an integral part of the body's defence mechanism both against infection and against cancerous change. Their job is to make antibodies which are specific chemicals which fight invading organisms such as bacteria and viruses.

Like white cells, plasma cells show marked proliferation during their naturally rapid turnover time. This normal process of rapid turnover can sometimes merge into overproduction and subsequently to cancerous change. When this occurs, the cancerous change is known as multiple myeloma.

The second type of cancer closely related to the leukaemias is a group of cancers known as the lymphomas, a particular form of which is known as Hodgkin's disease. These manifest themselves as an abnormal proliferation of lymphocytes which are found both in the blood and in the lymph nodes.

What causes leukaemias and lymphomas?

First, let us look at the leukaemias. Although there is no evidence of a direct hereditary factor in leukaemia there are indications that the disease is, in part, a hereditary phenomenon. In chronic myeloid leukaemia and some forms of acute leukaemia specific abnormalities can be seen in the chromosomes.

Viruses have also been implicated – although no specific virus has, as yet, been isolated in human leukaemias, viruses have definitely been shown to produce leukaemia in mice. Recently, too, sufferers with AIDS – a known viral infection – have been found to show evidence of leukaemic changes in their blood.

One definite cause of leukaemia is ionizing radiation evidenced most vividly after the dropping of the atomic bombs on Japan at the end of the Second World War. Acute leukaemia also developed in some patients who had been taking the anti-arthritic drug, phenylbutazone, which has now been withdrawn.

The cause of the lymphomas is unknown, apart from one very important exception. There is a particularly rare form of the disease known as the Burkitt tumour, named after the surgeon who both recognized and was able to suggest the possible cause of this tumour. While working in Africa, Burkitt noted that this particular tumour – which affects the lymph nodes, particularly those in the head and the neck – occurred in children, normally under the age of 15 years. More importantly, he noted that the tumours occurred in certain moist tropical areas at a particular altitude. He suggested that a virus could be responsible and, in 1964, two pathologists, Epstein and Barr, were able to isolate a virus, known as the Epstein Barr Virus, which, it is thought, may be responsible for the disease. This is one of the few instances where a virus can possibly be incriminated as causing cancer in humans. Whether or not the other lymphomas are caused by a virus, however, remains a matter for speculation.

What are the symptoms of acute leukaemia?

Acute leukaemia is seen both in children and adults.

I shall begin by describing the symptoms of acute leukaemia in children, though I must emphasize that these symptoms are non-specific and do not necessarily mean that any child with such symptoms has the disease. However, these symptoms should not be ignored and must be assessed by your doctor.

In the initial phases symptoms of acute leukaemia can pass unnoticed for it is difficult for many children – especially younger children – to say exactly what they are feeling. A child suffering from acute leukemia may appear listless and irritable, becoming tired rather more easily than usual, and lacking his normal energy. Head pains, limb pains and abdominal pains may all be experienced, and there will often be a number of visits to the surgery for infections that do not appear to be responding to antibiotics. Such symptoms are, of course, common in all children – especially young children. However, there are two symptoms which are particularly important and should not be overlooked. All children, at some time or another, knock themselves with resulting bruises. But if bruises appear with only slight evidence of trauma, this should be taken as a warning sign. A tendency to bleed, especially from oral areas such as lips and gums should also be treated seriously. When the child is taken to the doctor, enlarged lymph nodes and an enlarged spleen may be discovered.

In adults the following are characteristic symptoms and signs of acute leukaemia though again these are not specific to leukaemias. The patient may have been feeling generally unwell and a bit 'off colour' for a month or so. Often there may have been a flu-like illness that has never quite cleared up. Over the next few weeks he may have noticed, or may have been told by friends or relatives, that he looks paler than usual. He may have noticed that he is getting nose bleeds, that small cuts are bleeding rather more than usual and are taking much longer to heal. Slight breathlessness may have been experienced after what used to be considered mild exercise. Excessive tiredness may also be a feature of the disease, as are easy bruising and mouth ulcers that bleed easily. In addition, there may be a history of recurrent infection as well as infections not responding to antibiotic therapy. On examination, the doctor may find that the patient has an enlarged liver and spleen together with evidence of prominent lymph nodes. The reasons for these signs and symptoms, both in children and adults, is as follows. Acute leukaemia causes a reduction in platelets that causes the easy bruising and bleeding. A reduction in red cells (known as anaemia) is responsible for the feeling of tiredness and breathlessness, while the reduction in white cells is responsible for the body's inability to cope with infection.

The diagnosis of acute leukaemia is by a simple blood test, with the leukaemia cells being seen in the blood.

What are the symptoms of chronic leukaemia?

The chronic leukaemias are seen solely in adults. The two forms of the disease, chronic myeloid and chronic lymphatic leukaemia, can both occur in a very insidious manner. Again symptoms result from the malfunctioning of the body's white cells, red cells and platelets. They can develop over many months and, at first, appear quite innocuous. Fatigue and tiredness can be the first signs; also breathlessness on doing tasks that would normally be done without too much effort. These may be followed by other symptoms such as abnormal sweating, loss of appetite and weight, and itching. Nose bleeds and easy bruising together with abdominal discomfort tend to be late features of the disease. The symptoms of chronic lymphatic leukaemia can be very similar to those of chronic myeloid leukaemia though usually easy bruising and bleeding tend not to be a feature. Swollen lymph nodes may be prominent with infections, taking some time to clear up.

Chronic lymphatic leukaemia is considered to be the most benign form of leukaemia. It is seen most commonly in elderly people and tends to run a very low-key and protracted course. In some cases it is so benign that treatment is not required.

What are the symptoms of multiple myeloma?

Multiple myeloma occurs when there is a proliferation of plasma cells which are responsible for antibody production. The problem tends to occur in people in their mid-fifties and sixties.

The predominant symptom is bone pain, mainly in the back and in the ribs. This pain may be due to a pathological fracture that occurs when the bone becomes weakened by the disease process and eventually breaks under the strain. When this happens in the back, it is referred to as vertebral collapse.

Other symptoms of the disease are somewhat more nebulous. The function of plasma cells is to produce antibodies. Cancerous plasma cells do not produce antibodies of the quality needed to fight infection, with the result that recurrent infections can occur.

With the uncontrolled proliferation of plasma cells in the bone marrow the normal growth of red cells, white cells and platelets is affected. As a consequence tiredness, breathlessness, easy bruising and nose bleeds may be experienced. In some patients, kidney failure becomes a prominent feature. This is because the abnormally developing plasma cells produce a protein known as Bence Jones protein which accumulates in the kidneys, damaging their filtering apparatus. Consequently, the body's toxic wastes accumulate causing uraemia and high blood pressure.

What are the symptoms of Hodgkin's disease and lymphomas?

In Hodgkin's disease, cancerous change occurs in the lymphocytes, which are predominantly produced in the body's lymph nodes. It is not unsurprising, therefore, that the common symptom that heralds this problem is a swelling of the lymph nodes. This swelling is characteristically painless. The lymph nodes that are most commonly affected are in the neck, in the groin and in the axilla (armpit). Lymph nodes deeper within the body also swell, but cannot be felt. As well as the painless enlargement of lymph nodes there may be tiredness, lethargy and loss of weight.

Other characteristic features of Hodgkin's disease are an increased tendency to sweat – especially at night – and itching.

Lymphomas other than Hodgkin's disease may have very similar symptoms, but differ in that their disease process is not exclusively confined to the lymph nodes – other areas of the body can also be affected, including the bone marrow, the spleen and the liver.

How are the symptoms of leukemia investigated?

The initial test will normally be a simple blood test done by your GP. Under most circumstances, the haematology laboratory will, by looking at your blood cells, be able to confirm whether a blood disorder is present but before a definite diagnosis can be made, a bone marrow test will have to be performed. This may be done on an outpatients basis but is often done in hospital, where, if the diagnosis of leukaemia is confirmed, it is combined with the commencement of treatment.

The object of a bone marrow test is to acquire samples of the bone marrow so that the particular form of leukaemia can be precisely identified – this will have an important bearing on subsequent treatment.

Samples of bone marrow may be taken from the sternum (chest bone) or from the iliac crest, which is part of the hip bone. Following a local anaesthetic, a needle is passed through the bone to the central marrow cavity. Bone marrow cells are then removed through the needle and are spread out on a glass slide. This will then be sent to the haematology laboratory, where, by identifying which particular stem cell appears to be showing cancerous change, the precise form of the leukaemia or myeloma can be established.

As far as Hodgkin's disease and lymphomas are concerned, the investigations are rather more exhaustive, since these investigations are used not simply to establish the diagnosis, but also to establish how advanced the disease is, how far it has spread and the exact stage that it has reached.

Details of the staging of these diseases is beyond the scope of this book but I will just mention them in general terms. As you will recall, Hodgkin's disease is a cancerous disease of the lymph nodes.

The tests will centre around the extent to which the groups of lymph nodes throughout the body have been involved. The stages of Hodgkin's disease are as follows.

Stage 1 is represented by the involvement of a single group of lymph nodes, anywhere in the body. The second stage describes two or more involved groups of lymph nodes but stipulates that these should together lie on the same side of the diaphragm.

The third stage of Hodgkin's disease is where lymph nodes are involved on both sides of the diaphragm, and the fourth and most serious stage of the disease is reached when not only the lymph nodes are involved but when cancerous lymphocytes have invaded other structures such as the liver and bones.

There are a number of investigative techniques which are used to stage Hodgkin's disease. Blood tests and bone marrow investigations are done routinely. Radiological investigations usually follow. These will include ordinary X-rays of the chest, abdomen and bones. In addition, a specialized radiological investigation called a lymphangiogram will be done. In the procedure, a radio-opaque dye is injected into the lymphatic system and subsequent X-rays will show the dye collecting in the relevant groups of affected lymph nodes.

Recently CAT scanning (p.35) as well as other, non-radiological techniques such as ultrasound scanning, liver scanning and bone scanning have also been used.

An abdominal operation called a laparotomy is sometimes required, which involves looking into the abdomen and seeing directly whether or not the lymph nodes, spleen and liver are affected. The spleen and certain specimen lymph nodes are removed and the liver is biopsied.

Microscopic examination will then reveal whether or not these tissues have been infiltrated by cancerous lymphocytes.

How is acute leukaemia treated?

Acute leukaemia is one of the more common forms of cancers in children. Over the past two decades, the treatment of this cancer in children has undergone a revolution and from being a uniformly fatal illness it is now a condition that can both be brought under control and, in certain cases, be kept in remission for considerable lengths of time. Indeed, many centres have figures to show that up to half of all children treated can be said to be cured. The mainstay of treatment is chemotherapy aided by radiotherapy. Children are now, wherever possible, treated in special centres for children's cancers. The broad outlines of the treatment are threefold. The first stage is known as remission induction. The object of this is to eliminate all cancerous cells from the child's body. Then, once remission has been induced, radiotherapy (see pp.45-47) is given to the central nervous system (the brain and the spinal cord) – a completely painless procedure. Finally, maintenance therapy, involving the long-term treatment of the child, is started.

Remission induction is always started on an in-patient basis. This is not because the drugs are difficult to administer but because, while they are being given and are having their effects, some children will be prone to infection or at risk from bleeding. Once remission has been induced and radiotherapy has been given the child will be allowed home and will normally be treated on an outpatients basis. The child now enters the phase of remission maintenance. The drugs for this are given orally. Outpatient visits will be required at regular intervals so that investigations such as blood tests and bone marrow sampling can be done to check that the leukaemic cells are not beginning to return.

While receiving remission maintenance therapy any child who shows the slightest evidence of infection should be seen immediately so that the infection can be treated. Remission maintenance therapy, in some cases, may be stopped altogether.

However, there is always a possibility of relapse, in which case remission induction therapy is recommenced. Once the relapse is under control remission maintenance therapy is then continued. More recently, bone marrow transplants have been used with success in the more serious cases of childhood leukaemia.

The treatment of adult acute leukaemias is similar to the approach taken in children. The adult sufferer is sometimes physically in much worse condition than a child. Because of this, before remission induction therapy can be started, any problems of anaemia, bleeding and infections together with liver and kidney failure have to be stabilized and corrected. Once these problems are under control, remission induction therapy is commenced. The treatment takes the form of chemotherapy and can be given on an in-patient basis. It will require careful monitoring. Not only does the patient have to be watched for signs of increasing anaemia or recurring infections, but also for possible adverse side-effects from the drugs used to induce remission, which are necessarily powerful. These include vomiting and feelings of marked weakness – a situation that sometimes necessitates intravenous feeding – the sort of problems that require good general nursing care.

Once remission has been induced the patient will be allowed to go home and will be treated on an outpatient basis. This treatment is known as remission maintenance therapy, and consists of drugs, normally taken orally.

Routine blood tests and bone marrow samples are very important as a means of continually assessing whether the disease is recurring and if the drugs are doing more harm than good.

How are chronic leukaemias treated?

There are two basic forms of chronic leukaemia: chronic myeloid leukaemia and chronic lymphatic leukaemia.

Let us look at the treatment of chronic myeloid leukaemia first. The first line of therapy in this disease is chemotherapy, which is given on an outpatient basis. A commonly used drug in the treatment is busulphan, though patients taking this medication must have regular blood tests, since there is a thin dividing line between the drug's action of eradicating the cancerous white cells and destroying normal blood cells. Remission can last for long periods.

One of the prominent diagnostic features of chronic myeloid leukaemia is enlargement of both the liver and the spleen. Sometimes the spleen can grow to an enormous size causing abdominal discomfort. If this occurs an operation to remove the spleen (splenectomy) may be necessary. Recently, in certain cases, bone marrow transplants have been used with success in younger patients with this condition.

Chronic lymphatic leukaemia is normally the most benign form of leukaemia and in some very elderly patients will require no active treatment. Blood testing to ensure that the level of lymphocytes remains at a safe level is often all that is needed. In patients for whom treatment *is* necessary, chemotherapy is the mainstay of treatment. This treatment is taken orally and on an outpatient basis.

One of the reasons for not treating patients – especially the elderly – with this condition is that sometimes the bone marrow begins to fail of its own accord and this process can be accelerated by these chemotherapeutic agents.

How is multiple myeloma treated?

The mainstay of therapy for this condition is chemotherapy. The two drugs most commonly used are melphalan and cyclophosphamide, though the steroid preparation, prednisolone, is also administered. All these drugs adversely affect the plasma cells that are proliferating in the bone marrow.

Another important aspect of the treatment of multiple myeloma is the need to tackle the secondary effects of this disease, especially as they relate to bone. It is important to be mobile. Lying in bed will lead to demineralization of bones, which contributes to the further weakening of already weakened bones. This process, together with the effects of metastases, can lead to pathological fractures.

Radiotherapy to these areas greatly reduces the pain that arises from these sites.

Multiple myeloma, together with these secondary effects, causes the functions of the bone marrow to be compromised. This means that the consequent anaemia and the lowered platelet content of the blood will often have to be corrected by blood and platelet transfusion.

Infections are not uncommon and have to be treated vigorously. In cases where the kidney is affected, measures must be taken to prevent renal failure.

How are Hodgkin's disease and lymphomas treated?

The two mainstays of therapy are radiation treatment and chemotherapy. When I discussed the diagnosis of Hodgkin's disease (see p.119) I emphasized the importance of staging. It is on the basis of this that the various types of treatment are given. Stages 1 and 2 of the condition are treated by radiotherapy supplemented by chemotherapy but in the more advanced stages, 3 and 4, the mainstay of treatment will be chemotherapy. A series of drugs may be used, such treatment being known as combination therapy (see Drug Glossary, pp.156-159).

Hodgkin's disease is one of the few cancers to respond extremely well to treatment. In many instances those with this disease will go into complete remission for many years. This puts the treatment of Hodgkin's disease very much in the vanguard of cancer therapy.

With the lymphomas, radiotherapy and chemotherapy are the mainstays of treatment. Some lymphomas are not confined to lymph nodes but may be widely spread throughout the various tissues of the body. In these cases, specific radiotherapy treatment will be difficult, and chemotherapy, in the form of combination therapy, will give the best chances of remission.

What is cancer of the urinary system?

This can take the form of cancer of the bladder or cancer of the kidney.

What are the symptoms of kidney and bladder cancer?

The features of kidney cancer and bladder cancer can be very similar, the main difference being that the symptoms of kidney cancer often occur late in the disease.

The most important symptom of both bladder cancer and kidney cancer is blood in the urine; this is known as haematuria. Other symptoms may include raised temperature, fever and night sweats. An important symptom of bladder cancer is frequency, which means the need to pass urine more often than usual. Sometimes, too, passing urine may be painful, a condition known as dysuria.

Kidney cancer often causes pain in the loin. In some cases of the disease a hormone called parathyroid hormone is produced. Excess amounts of this hormone cause nausea and sometimes vomiting as well as a need to drink abnormal quantities of water.

As is often the case with cancer symptoms, however, these are not specific for either bladder cancer or kidney cancer. For example, blood in the urine or pain on passing urine are most commonly due to infection of the urinary system, while drinking excessive amounts of water and passing excessive amounts of urine may be the initial symptoms of diabetes mellitus. The simple message is, if you have these symptoms go to your doctor and get them checked out.

What causes bladder cancer and kidney cancer?

Bladder cancers were one of the first cancers to be directly implicated as being caused by an industrial process; in the nineteenth century, they were found in workers in the dye industry.

This problem has now been eliminated, though another cause of the disease – chronic irritation of the bladder lining by a small, worm-like microbe called a schistosoma – is prevalent in the Middle East. This microbe lives and multiples within the bladder, initiating a chronic inflammation of the bladder wall. Artificial sweeteners and smoking have also been incriminated, but there is no hard evidence to support these claims.

The cause of cancer of the kidney is unknown, though industrial processes that involve the use of cadmium have been implicated.

How are these cancers investigated?

The most common and most important sign of both bladder cancer and kidney cancer is haematuria (blood in the urine). If the haematuria is not due to an infection your GP will arrange for you to see a urologist (a surgeon who specializes in disorders of the urinary system). The urologist will feel the lower parts of your abdomen, to detect any pelvic swellings which might indicate spread of a bladder cancer, and also your loin, for swellings that might indicate kidney cancer. He will then order routine X-rays of both your chest and abdomen and also an intravenous pyelogram (see p.34). However, by far and away the most important investigation will be a cystoscopy, which will involve an overnight stay in hospital. This test is normally done under general anaesthetic, although sometimes epidural anaethesia, which numbs the lower half of the body, is used. Cystoscopy involves passing a cystoscope (a hollow steel tube, within which is a light source) through the urethra and into the bladder, thus allowing the surgeon direct visualization of the bladder lining. In this way, areas of cancerous change can be both examined and biopsied. If, following cystoscopy, no cancer is found in the bladder, the kidney will be investigated for cancerous change. Ultrasound examination of a suspicious lesion in or around the kidney can help towards a definitive diagnosis. The most useful test is that of the CAT scan (see p.35), which allows for detailed X-ray assessment of any lesions in or around the kidney.

How is bladder cancer treated?

Treatment of bladder cancer depends on the stage of the disease when it is first discovered. In the earliest stages of the disease, the cancer will appear as a warty growth on the internal lining of the bladder, known as a papillary carcinoma. The next main stage is reached when the cancer extends into the bladder wall to involve the muscle in this wall. Finally, the most advanced stage is when the cancer has extended beyond the bladder wall and encroaches on other organs in the pelvis. All these stages can be subdivided further by assessing the spread of the cancer to the local lymph nodes.

In the earliest stage of bladder cancer the growth can normally be removed at the initial cystoscopy, by simply burning the papillary carcinoma from the bladder wall with a diathermy probe, which is introduced into the cystoscope. This procedure is often curative in itself, though it will be necessary to have repeat cystoscopy examinations because the rate of recurrence of these cancers is quite high.

In addition to this surgical treatment, external or internal radiotherapy can be given (see pp.45-47). Internal radiotherapy in this case will involve introducing a radioactive compound into the bladder which irradiates all suspicious areas of the bladder lining. The radioactive solution is subsequently washed out of the bladder.

For the intermediate stages of bladder cancer the part of the bladder which contains the cancer is surgically removed. Following this, radiotherapy is given either externally or internally.

In some centres, chemotherapy may be given in the form of a solution directly introduced into the bladder. Repeat cystoscopies will be required to detect and treat recurrences. In the late stages of bladder cancer there is normally no alternative but to remove the bladder completely, a procedure which may be followed by both radiotherapy and chemotherapy.

Removal of the bladder clearly presents a problem. The bladder is responsible for collecting the urine that is produced by the kidneys, and then discharging it in the urethra. If the bladder is removed, an artificial bladder has to be surgically made. In the operation, the surgeon selects a segment of the small bowel known as the ileum. Freeing this piece of ileum from the remainder of the small intestine, he closes off one end, making it into a small pouch, then brings the open end through the abdominal wall, allowing it to open to the exterior, to form a stoma. He will then take the ureters (the tubes that carry the urine from the kidney to the bladder) and transplant them into the ileal pouch that he has fashioned (which is known as an ileal conduit). In this way the kidneys excrete their urine into this artificial bladder. The urine is collected by a special ostomy bag which covers the external ileal conduit.

At night time, to prevent overflow from the ostomy bag, a 'two-way' valve at its base can be connected to a drainage tube that can gradually collect the night's urinary output. This avoids the problem of having to get up during the night to empty the ostomy bag. Normally the bag has to be emptied every three or four hours, the valve at the bottom of the bag facilitating this emptying routine.

Patients with ileal conduits need not modify their diets.

How is kidney cancer treated?

The mainstay of kidney cancer treatment is surgery. This involves a nephrectomy (removal of the diseased kidney).

Surprisingly, this does not affect the body's renal function, the remaining kidney being able to cope with the excretory functions previously performed by its partner. Local external radiotherapy will sometimes be given following the operation.

What is cancer of the testicle?

The chief sign of testicular cancer is a swelling in one testicle. Usually the swelling is painless and hard; a tender swelling is more likely to be due to an infection of the testicle rather than cancer.

Men in their thirties and forties are particularly prone to this form of cancer and its cause is unknown, though there is one very important predisposing factor known as maldescent of the testes.

During the course of normal development, the testicles, which begin life in the abdomen, pass from the abdomen and through the pelvis into the scrotum.

Maldescent of the testicles refers to any interruption of this normal progression of the testicles from the abdomen to the scrotum, though exactly why cancer should develop more commonly in such testicles is not known.

If you have a testicular swelling you will be referred to a urologist (a surgeon who specializes in disease of the urinary system and the genitals).

After an initial examination, the urologist will normally advise surgical exploration of the testicular swelling. This will involve having an operation under general anaesthesia. If the surgeon finds the swelling to be cancerous, he will perform an orchidectomy (removal of the testicle).

Further tests to see if the cancer has spread outside the testicle will include lymphangiography, together with a CAT scan (see p.35).

With the results of these investigations the urologist will then be able to stage the tumour. The two most common malignant tumours of the testicle are known as seminoma and teratoma. Both follow the same pattern of development. In the early stages of the disease the cancer will be restricted to the testicular tissue. The second stage is where spread has occurred to lymph nodes lying in the abdomen known as the retroperitoneal nodes. The third and most advanced stage is where cancer metastases have spread beyond these nodes to other structures such as the liver, lungs or bones.

How is cancer of the testicle treated?

The first stage is orchidectomy (surgical removal of the testicle). Further treatment depends on the type of testicular cancer and the stage to which it has spread through the body. With seminomas, external radiotherapy will be given to the retroperitoneal lymph nodes. With teratomas the mainstay of treatment is chemotherapy, though some centres will advise radiotherapy to the retroperitoneal nodes (in the USA some surgeons acutally advise surgical removal of these nodes). The chemotherapy is given in the form of combination therapy and this necessarily has to be done on an in-patient basis.

What is cancer of the ovary?

Cancer of the ovary describes various malignant changes within the ovarian tissue. These can either be cystic or solid in nature.

The reason why cancer arises in the ovary is unknown. In Japanese women living in Japan, the incidence of ovarian cancer is low, while in immigrant Japanese women living in the USA, the incidence of this cancer approximates to the norm for American women. This suggests that environmental causes may have a role to play.

Evidence for a genetic cause comes from the association of a relatively higher incidence of ovarian cancer in those women of blood group A.

One of the problems in diagnosing cancer of the ovary is that it gives little in the way of symptoms until, in some cases, it is very large and advanced. Symptoms that can be due to ovarian cancers are usually non-specific, and include weight loss, loss of appetite, tiredness, feelings of abdominal fullness, abdominal distention, intermittent abdominal pain, slight changes in bowel habit and changes in urinary habit. It is precisely because of the vagueness of the symptoms that many ovarian cancers tend to be diagnosed late.

As a consequence, they have often spread beyond the ovary and with this spread there is the increased difficulty in treating both the primary cancer and the metastases. The diagnosis of an ovarian swelling, whether benign or malignant, can be made on pelvic examination.

It is for this reason that it has been suggested that all women, when they go for their routine cervical smear, should also have a pelvic examination so that any ovarian swellings may be detected. If this procedure were routine, many more ovarian cancers would be detected earlier in their development and so would be more easily treated. It has recently been suggested that ultrasound screening for ovarian cancer should be routinely available for all women.

When you are referred to a gynaecologist he will confirm the diagnosis of an ovarian swelling but, like your general practitioner, will not be in a position to state whether or not the tumour is benign or malignant. Further tests, including a CAT scan (see p.35) and possibly an ultrasound examination will be required.

An exploratory abdominal operation under general anaesthesia will then follow so that the swelling may be directly visualized. This may take the form of a laparoscopy, a procedure that involves the use of an instrument called a laproscope to directly visualize the pelvic organs without having to make a large abdominal incision. If a suspicious ovarian growth is seen the consultant will then proceed to a formal abdominal operation if this is indicated (see below).

How is cancer of the ovary treated?

Surgery is the treatment of choice. If cancer is found in one ovary, both ovaries will probably have to be removed. This is because, in a certain percentage of cases, on microscopic examination, evidence of early cancerous change in the other ovary may be found.

The operation to remove both ovaries is known as bilateral oophorectomy. It is normally combined with a total hysterectomy – the whole operation sometimes being referred to as a pelvic clearance operation.

The removal of the ovaries means that the source of the hormone oestrogen is removed. This may present problems in pre-menopausal women but these can be solved by hormone replacement therapy.

Once the ovarian cancer has been removed the gynaecologist will then make a careful search throughout the abdomen for signs of cancerous spread from the primary tumour. In this way, the staging (assessment of the amount of spread of the tumour) can be established.

Subsequent therapy will depend upon this initial staging process. Stage 1 is when cancerous tissue is seen only in either one or other ovary. Stage 2 refers to a spread limited to the immediate vicinity of the ovaries – in other words in the pelvis. Stage 3 is when the cancer has spread out of the pelvis to involve abdominal structures such as the lymph nodes and the large and small bowel. In the fourth and most serious stage the cancer has spread throughout the abdomen, involving the liver, and may well have spread into the chest. Treatment following surgery is based upon this staging. For those women who are found to be at Stage 1, following surgery, if the cancer in the ovary was at an early stage of development, no further treatment is necessary.

However, normally surgery will be followed by radiotherapy. Those patients with Stage 2 cancer, following surgery, will normally have radiation therapy to both their pelvis and their abdomen. For those patients with the more advanced stages of ovarian cancer – Stages 3 and 4 – surgery is followed by radiation therapy to both the pelvis and abdomen. In addition, chemotherapy is also given in the form known as combination therapy (see Drug Glossary pp.156-159).

Psychological and social aspects

What are the psychological problems associated with a diagnosis of cancer?

This is a difficult question to answer. Not only are there many forms of cancer to take into account but, most importantly, each cancer sufferer is an individual. Such a person must cope with the emotional impact of being told that he has cancer as well as all the normal psychological problems that we all face at different times in our lives.

In view of the vast scope of this subject I am going to take one particular form of cancer, breast cancer, and discuss the psychological problems that may emerge as a result of developing this particular form of the disease. Although I shall be only talking about one type of cancer, however, I must emphasize that many of the underlying psychological problems with this disease are common to all cancers.

A particularly important point that I should like to make, right from the start, is that although breast cancer is an individual problem, the person concerned is also normally a member of a family or social grouping. When discussing psychological implications of cancer, it is important to take this into account and to consider the psychological impact on both the individual and her family.

So, let us take the case of a woman who, quite correctly, is conducting a routine self-examination of her breast. She comes across what she thinks is a breast lump which she knows could possibly be a sign of cancer. The fact that she is examining her breasts at all means that she is aware of the risks of breast cancer and probably has a basic knowledge of what the disease can entail. Her thought processes will naturally think along the lines of mastectomy. It is quite natural, at this stage, for there to be an immediate and an intense emotional response. This often manifests itself as a denial of the symptom – not in the sense of consciously denying that the lump is there but, rather, in the sense of assuming that it is transient, a temporary problem that will go away. Such a denial response may often be the initial reaction of both the patient and her partner. This can be a dangerous psychological period because denial of the lump may lead to a delay in seeking treatment. Again, this is perfectly natural. The patient and her family, if she has confided in them, may mutually reassure each other that the symptom is only temporary, that it will go away. Both, however, while unable to verbalize their feelings, will nevertheless be shocked by the discovery of the breast lump. And this shock can cause confusion as to what to do. This will manifest itself as indecision about whether or not to act upon the symptoms immediately.

Alternatively, there may be a completely different psychological response to the discovery of a breast lump, and a state resembling an acute anxiety reaction can occur, where the patient, on discovering a breast lump, immediately goes to her doctor. This acute anxiety reaction is often fuelled by the natural worry of relatives and friends. This complex series of psychological reactions will be understood by the GP who will realize that there may be further emotional difficulties as his patient passes through the various stages of investigation and treatment.

The next major psychological hurdle centres around the assessment of the breast lump by the surgeon and the taking of the biopsy. Waiting for the results of the biopsy tests is inevitably a period of great stress for both the patient and her family. Now that the initial symptom can no longer be denied, now that she knows that the symptom, the breast lump, is 'real' and is being investigated, the patient's initial anxieties about mastectomy followed by a fear of possible terminal illness will become much more sharply focused. At the same time the family will, to a certain extent, feel in a helpless situation. The natural uncertainty about what is taking place, together with future uncertainties, leaves them feeling unable to help the patient, which, in turn, can induce anxiety.

Once the diagnosis of breast cancer has been made and the patient is asked to come into the hospital for treatment, the psychological tension of both patient and family begins to rise. This, for the patient, is due to a number of factors – amongst them a sense of a loss of identity and helplessness and a feeling that she is losing control over her own destiny. This may manifest itself as resentment towards the doctors and nurses at the hospital as well as an ambivalence towards the proposed treatment. Such feelings almost certainly overlie an increasingly deep-seated anxiety as control over her life and body seem to be slipping away from her.

Similarly, her husband may feel that she is being taken away from him and her children may worry that they will lose their mother; that they are somehow being left alone to cope with a situation over which they have no control and the outcome of which is uncertain. Again, this psychological reaction can manifest itself as ambivalence or hostility towards the medical staff – a reaction that these professionals will understand and appreciate.

Once the decision to operate has been made, the anxiety of both patient and family will reach a peak. I must emphasize that the medical staff will be aware of the emotional stresses and strains both upon the patient and the patient's family during the pre-operative and operative period. Often, once treatment is successfully completed, a sense of guilt can worry some patients and their families when they look back and recall their uncharacteristic behaviour towards those who have helped them. Don't worry about this. As I have said, the medical and nursing teams are aware of these psychological conflicts and appreciate them for what they are – natural reactions to a very stressful situation.

Further and quite natural anxiety before a mastectomy operation is the fear of disfigurement, long-term loss of femininity and the uncertainties of future health; a fear of both the physical and the psychological unknown. As far as the family's psychological reactions to the operative period is concerned, the fears are centred not so much upon longer-term future problems such as terminal illness but, rather, upon the immediate problem, that of wife and mother getting successfully through the operation. For all the parties involved, there may also be the added anxieties of exclusion and loneliness – a feeling that strangers, in some way, are taking over and dominating their lives.

What are the psychological reactions of both the patient and the family following the operation?

After the operation, physical and psychological recovery begin. This can be a period of great psychological fluctuation for both patient and family. Initially, there may be relief that the operation is over, but when the operation site is dressed and the drainage tubes and the scar of the operation become visible, the physical absence of a breast may well emphasize the pre-operative fear of disfigurement. This is usually followed by a feeling that the treatment is going according to plan and hope begins to emerge with feelings that, although there will be some disfigurement, the cancer has been taken away, the cancer has been cured. Set against these optimistic psychological feelings is often a series of pessimistic psychological fears that the cancer may recur and that the operation has not completely cured the problem, that she may be faced with a long-term terminal illness. The patient may also fear her husband will no longer love her.

These two conflicting and fluctuating psychological states may give the impression of a contradictory post-operative psychological response. At times the patient may seem to be well, happy, and coping with the routine post-operative problems; at others she will seem tearful, resentful, angry, depressed and anxious, with episodes of smiling suddenly turning to tears.

After the operation, the family may go through a phase of psychological relief once they see that wife and mother is making an uncomplicated recovery. But this early reaction often reverts to anxiety as doubts about recurrence occur. These doubts, together with anger and frustration at the ongoing sense of helplessness, are often repressed, again sometimes manifesting themselves as an ambivalence in mood towards both patient and medical staff.

In particular, the husband may begin to contemplate whether or not sexual relations will be altered following his wife's discharge from hospital. He may even wonder at times if they will ever have sexual relations again. This may obviously be a particularly stressful thought for him.

What psychological problems can follow discharge from hospital?

Although the woman may be relieved to get home, the anxieties over coping with her mastectomy on her own may become more acute now that the nurses and doctors are not constantly present. Initial feelings of weakness and tiredness and an obvious inability to perform household tasks are inevitable and these feelings, superimposed upon all her other worries and fears, may leave her feeling inadequate, unable to cope and very lonely. She may feel that she will be a burden on her family for ever.

Problems may be compounded even further by the fact that she still needs treatment such as chemotherapy and radiotherapy. Radiotherapy in itself can be responsible for tiredness and depression, but chemotherapy may produce additional side-effects, including nausea, depression, hair loss and – inevitable, at this time – varying degrees of loss of libido, or sexual desire. All these problems can tend to reinforce the patient's fears that she is losing her independence, and is never going to get better. Similarly, the family – and the patient's husband, in particular – may not have fully appreciated at the time of the operation what these further forms of therapy would entail, and may feel angry that the operation has not been successful in itself; further treatment confirms previously held fears that the doctors were not able to cure the cancer with the operation. They had, in all probability, hoped that things would return to normal following the operation; instead things may in some ways appear worse after the operation with no obvious signs of getting better.

During this phase great psychological stresses and strains can be suffered by the family.

As far as the patient is concerned, anger may be very prominent. Anger at everybody, both doctors and family; anger at the realization that she has cancer. Why should *she* have developed cancer? Why was it *she* who had to undergo the operation and suffer the consequent loss of such an important symbol of her femininity? These are all natural reactions which may start to surface as the future begins to unfold, and may show themselves in all sorts of ways.

A common manifestation may be the avoidance of intimate sexual contact with her husband. She may dread him seeing her undressed and fear that he will reject her. Similarly, the husband, who may not understand or be aware of these psychological problems – seeing that, to all intents and purposes, his wife appears to be getting better – may naturally resent the ambivalence, or even anger she has directed towards him. He may feel rejected, and worry that the withdrawal of sexual favours in some way reflects upon his attitude for her. He may feel guilty about asking her to participate in sexual relations while she is coping with a life-threatening condition.

Under these circumstances it is terribly easy for communication to break down between husband and wife, and this is often a very great and real problem following mastectomy. In addition, this period of emotional instability within the family often coincides with long-term treatment such as radiotherapy and chemotherapy, which in themselves can prevent the patient from feeling both physically and psychologically better.

However, resolution of these problems will eventually occur. In the long term, once physical acceptance of mastectomy has been achieved and the effects of the radiotherapy and chemotherapy are seen to be beneficial, there is likely to be a return to the normal physical and psychological state that existed before the operation. Many of the patient's and the family's worries, fears and anxieties begin to evaporate, and the patient starts inwardly to accept the loss of her breast and begins to regain her sense of femininity. Her prosthesis or reconstructed breast no longer seems alien to her.

With new clothes her confidence begins to return, and she begins to reintegrate her body image, which has received a psychological battering, into her new self-image. She finds herself able to perform all her old tasks and she starts to feel that sexually she is becoming attractive once more and that her husband still loves and accepts her despite the loss of her breast.

As confidence begins to come back, family life starts to return to normal.

Husband and family finally accept that the treatment has worked and the long-term future is secure. The level of anxiety begins to quickly fall and although the mastectomy is never completely forgotten, normal family routines begin to replace the anxieties and problems that both the operation and the post-operative period posed.

There will obviously be episodes when anxieties resurface. This may often occur just before hospital outpatient appointments for follow-up and checks. Again, this psychological reaction is wholly understandable.

I hope that, having described the psychological problems surrounding the specific diagnosis and treatment of breast cancer, I have demonstrated that at each phase in the physical treatment programme there is a concomitant psychological phase that has to be borne separately by the patient and the patient's family. This, to a large extent, is true of most cancers and is the reason why cancer counselling is becoming an important part of cancer therapy in general.

How do I cope with a diagnosis of cancer?

Before answering this question I would like to emphasize a point that, I hope, has been apparent throughout this book. As you have read through the various sections two things should have become apparent to you. Firstly, although the precise nature of cancer is unknown, an enormous body of knowledge has accumulated and much is known about the basic scientific nature of cancer. Secondly, not only are there many different forms of cancer but some of these cancers grow slowly and, in some cases, take decades to develop. In addition, some cancers, while not entirely preventable, are certainly curable if their symptoms are acted upon immediately.

A diagnosis of cancer is not a death sentence and should never be regarded as such. Modern medicine can, to a large extent, palliate disease and give the cancer sufferer many years of normal active life. Many patients with cancer live a natural lifespan and commonly die as a result of an entirely different problem, such as a heart attack. It is essential to bear these facts in mind. Even while bearing these positive facts in mind, however, to be told that you have cancer will probably be one of the worst experiences in your life. I think that the root of this problem lies in the very word 'cancer'. Doctors know that some cancers are more serious than others and that to tell a patient that they have, for example, a rodent ulcer on their face (a curable skin cancer) is not a particularly serious message to have to give, because they know that the cancer can be completely eradicated and, in most circumstances, will not recur. On the other hand.

the patient, once he hears the word 'cancer' quite naturally reacts in a completely different way because of the word and all the symbolism that it conjures up in the imagination. Most patients are unlikely to know if their particular cancer is one of the less serious cancers. To most patients, cancer is cancer. To a patient who has a rodent ulcer this cancer may seem to him exactly the same disease that affected his neighbour, who recently died of, say, lung cancer.

This underlines a particularly important principle; communication between the doctor, patient and patient's family must be effective. If the word cancer is used then it mustn't simply be allowed to hang in the air without explanation. If a doctor tells a patient that he has cancer then a full explanation must follow. The doctor must explain, in intelligible terms, the basic nature of the particular cancer, how it will be investigated, and how long this will take; the method and length of treatment and any side-effects that may occur; the length of convalescence time that will be needed, and whether or not returning to a former job or occupation is a viable possibility.

The patient must, at the very outset, be given a simple explanation of what his particular cancer is, and the effects that it might have on his subsequent life.

In this respect, the example that I have chosen when talking about a less serious form of cancer (the rodent ulcer, a skin cancer) represents a medical dilemma. As I have pointed out, this is a particularly innocuous form of cancer that can be easily treated and is not life-threatening. In other words, although technically it is a cancer it does not behave or develop in the same way as other, more serious cancers. The dilemma arises when the doctor wonders if he should use the word 'cancer' when telling his patient that he has a rodent ulcer of his skin. Should he tell his patient that he has an 'ulcer' on his skin and then deliberately avoid using the word cancer? Such a decision is obviously taken with the patient's interest in mind. The doctor will be well aware of the connotation that the word cancer has and, not wishing to distress his patient, may feel that it is unnecessary to burden him with all the psychological torment that this emotive word can arouse.

In certain circumstances this may be a valid attitude but, on the other hand, it does have its problems. To continue with my example of the rodent ulcer, in a very small percentage of patients this cancerous skin change can recur and, in exceptional circumstances, may develop into a rather more serious cancerous process. What will happen in those very few cases where patients who have been led to believe that their skin lesion was not cancerous, subsequently discover that not only was the lesion cancerous but the doctor, for whatever well-intentioned motives, kept this information from them? Understandably, they will feel that they have been deceived. How can they possibly trust their doctor in the future? Will what he tells them be true or not? Will all doctors, in the future, withhold information and not tell the truth? It is understandable that such patients can have little faith in doctors and still less faith and trust in their treatments. This is how trust and communication between doctor and patient can break down.

But this is not the end of the story. It can often come as a considerable shock to a family to discover that, all along, the problem has been cancer when they were led to believe otherwise. Such a situation will also lead to a breakdown of trust and communication between the doctor and the patient's family. The family members subsequently find it hard to trust that particular doctor and doctors, in general, and when they, in turn, become ill, will wonder if they are being told the truth by their doctors.

This problem highlights two very important principles: if a patient has cancer, in most circumstances, he and his family should be told. At the same time, once the word cancer has been used, then its full implications should be thoroughly discussed and explained.

Informed communication between doctor, the patient and the patient's family will build a bridge of trust, and this bridge will be important for subsequent treatment. If a patient and his family trust their doctor this, alone, goes a long way to the eventual success of any treatment. This sense of trust will also allow the patient and his family to feel that the doctor and any member of his medical team is always approachable.

Doctors can in some circumstances be bad communicators, but such communication problems should not be allowed to persist. There are a number of ways of establishing good rapport between all parties. When you are told by your consultant that you have cancer he should, as I have just stated, tell you in simple terms the exact nature of the problem and how he proposes to treat you, together with the long-term outlook. If this does not happen, and you are confused or left wondering exactly what has been said or if you want a particular aspect or point emphasized or explained again, then do not hesitate to ask him directly. I know this is easier said than done. The realization that you have a diagnosis of cancer can initially be overwhelming. You may simply not be in a position to verbalize your anxieties and fears. It may only be after you have left the hospital that the full impact of what you have been told begins to be fully appreciated.

Finding the words for further questions to the consultant who has just given you this bad news is often, quite naturally, impossible. In addition, this may well be the first time that you will have met your consultant and you may have difficulty in talking to a stranger. Even if you do manage to ask questions at this first consultation, the answers that you receive may not be fully understood. Do ask questions, nevertheless, at this initial meeting. Your consultant will be fully aware of the strains and pressures that have immediately been put on you and will always do his best to explain any doubts and questions that have arisen in your mind. Remember, too, this will not be the only time you meet your consultant – there will be many other opportunities to ask him these questions. Between the time of your first consultation and your subsequent appointment, therefore, decide which questions you would like answered, and write them down on a piece of paper. Talk about any aspects of your cancer that are worrying you with friends and relatives. They may well have useful suggestions for questions that you can ask. Another useful tip is to be accompanied to the hospital by a friend or relative who can sit with you when the consultant is talking to you. This can have two advantages. Firstly, they may help you remember the questions you wanted to ask your consultant. Secondly, they also will hear what your consultant said to you about your particular problem. In one's anxiety about a particular problem, it is often easy to mishear or misinterpret what has been said. If someone else has been a party to the conversation then contentious points can be discussed at leisure when you are back in the comfort of your own home.

There is another, equally important avenue of acquiring knowledge about your particular condition. Following your appointment at the hospital, your consultant will always write a letter to your GP stating the exact nature of the diagnosis, the results of all the investigations and the way in which he proposes to treat you. Ring up the surgery and speak to the receptionist. Ask if your doctor has received a letter from the consultant. When this letter has been received, ask to see your GP. Doctors are only too glad to provide this service. Remember, your GP knows you. He knows how best to explain things to you. It is possible that the consultant, in an effort to communicate with you, may have used some misleading terms. Your doctor, knowing you, will not have this problem. With the consultant's letter in front of him, he will be able to explain to you, in terms that he knows you will understand, exactly what is going on.

You will inevitably be very much more at ease with your own doctor and will probably find it easier to ask him the questions that you might have found rather more difficult to ask a strange consultant. Even if you feel that your visit to the hospital and the subsequent conversation with the consultant has been fairly comprehensive, therefore, I would still advise that you go to your GP. He will be interested to see you, to find out how you are coping with the diagnosis of cancer and if, in any way, he can help. Remember, he will be at your side through all stages of treatment and rehabilitation and the sooner he gets to grips with your problem the better. After all, you are his patient. He has brought the consultant in to treat you.

So, to summarize. The first stage in coping with a diagnosis of cancer is to discuss the problem with as many people as possible: your consultant at the hospital, your friends, your relatives and your GP. Communication is all important. The more you talk about your cancer the more you will understand about it. The more you understand about your cancer the more you will appreciate why you are receiving particular treatments.

Active involvement at all stages of diagnosis, investigations and treatment will not only allay your fear but will enable you to concentrate your mind on the positive aspects of the problem, coming through the treatment in the best possible shape with a positive attitude towards the future.

Having said all this, however, don't feel that you have to take the total burden of your cancer completely on your own shoulders. Your doctors are responsible for looking after you through the various stages of investigation and treatment. It is their job to treat you as best they can and they certainly will. Keep an active interest in the investigations and treatment but let your doctors do the worrying for you. Let them cope with the technical problems.

Does cancer cause pain?

It is a common misconception that cancer automatically causes pain. Many cancers, even in their advanced stages, do not cause pain. The first important point to emphasize, therefore, is that just because you have cancer it does not necessarily mean to say that you will inevitably experience pain. Pain does accompany some cancers, but with modern techniques and therapies it can be controlled. If you are experiencing pain, therefore, report this to your doctor immediately.

Pain itself is a strange sensation and it is often difficult to describe, even to the extent of being very precise as to where the pain is coming from. Pain is also a very individual sensation, and different people will experience the same pain in different ways. In other words, some of us experience pain more easily than others. Pain can also be affected by psychological status. If morale is low and depression and anxiety are a problem then the sensation of pain is probably more pronounced. Inevitably, when discussing pain, all these general factors have to be taken into consideration.

There are various different causes of pain but I must emphasize that some of these are rare and that in many cancer patients severe, prolonged pain is never experienced.

What causes cancer pain?

There are many different causes of cancer pain and this is why different forms of pain treatment may have to be used at various times. One of the most common causes is cancerous infiltration of bone, normally in the form of metastases. Take, for example, the vertebral column. Pain here can arise from the fact that cancer has spread to the bone, but it can also be due to a weakening effect on the vertebral bodies causing what is known as vertebral collapse. Nerves, from the spinal cord, pass out through holes (foramina) in these vertebral bodies. A collapsed vertebral body may trap one or more of these nerves as they pass through the foramina, and this will cause pain.

Other ways in which metastases can cause pain is by causing what is termed a pathological fracture (a vertebral collapse is a form of pathological fracture). Here, the cancer spreads to a bone, for example in the leg, causing weakening of the bone. The bone is eventually unable to support the weight of the body, resulting in fracture of the bone with subsequent pain.

Cancers can also spread directly into nerves with self-evidently painful results, as well as weakness of muscles – a problem that may further compound the pain.

Pain may also be due to the effects of the primary tumour. In bowel cancer, for instance, the tumour may cause blockage of the intestines causing obstruction which manifests itself as abdominal pain.

All these are examples of pain caused by the cancer, itself; but there are still further causes of pain, which relate to the treatment of the cancer. For instance following surgery. Operations on the chest, head and neck can cause post-operative pain. If a limb has been amputated, pain may arise from the amputation site.

In some cases, radiotherapy may itself be the cause of pain. Occasionally, it may induce side-effects causing slight damage to tissues surrounding the field of radiation with pain coming from these damaged nerves and bones. Chemotherapy also sometimes causes painful problems because some chemotherapeutic agents can damage nerves.

On top of these causes of pain related to cancer, there are the normal pain problems experienced by everybody, and both these and a psychological lowering of morale can compound cancer pain.

How is cancer pain treated?

Before dealing with this particularly important question I would like to make a general point about pain therapy. I'd like to take the migraine headache as an illustrative example (though, of course, migraine headaches have *no* connection with cancer). The migraine headache is a particularly unpleasant form of pain. Some sufferers from this condition have to go to bed with the curtains drawn and remain like this for hours on end, such is the intensity of the pain. Migraine-sufferers often know when an attack is about to come on. They also know that if they take pain-relieving treatment before the migraine develops there will be a much greater chance of lessening the effects of the headache than if they take the tablets once the migraine has started. In other words, they anticipate the pain; they do not wait for it to begin.

Similarly, for cancer patients with pain the crucially important aim of pain control is to anticipate the pain and so keep it under control all the time. This may mean using strong pain-killing drugs on a regular basis but, in the case of cancer patients, the drugs are, in the main, non-addictive. With this basic principle in mind, let us look at some of the drugs that are available to combat cancer pain.

In the majority of cases, cancer pain is not a major problem and only a mild pain-killing tablet may have to be used. Drugs such as aspirin or paracetamol are excellent for this form of mild intermittent cancer pain.

If moderate pain is experienced (though what might be moderate pain to one person may well be mild pain to another), drugs such as codeine, distalgesic or DF118 are useful.

For more severe pain, stronger drugs must be used, amongst which are morphine and methadone.

As well as these pain-killing drugs, other drugs can lessen pain by directly relieving symptoms. When we discussed brain tumours I mentioned that expansion of the brain tissue caused by the tumour within the skull, was a cause of headache. Dexamethasone is a steroid drug which reduces this swelling, thus easing the pain of raised intracranial pressure. Similarly, pain due to compression of a nerve can often be relieved by the steroid drug prednisolone, while stomach symptoms will respond to drugs such as chlorpromazine and metoclopramide. Pain from infections can be greatly relieved with antibiotics.

Muscle spasms can also be the result of cancer either affecting the muscle directly or the nerves supplying those muscles. A muscle-relaxant such as valium can be of great value under these circumstances.

What are pain clinics?

Over the past few years, pain clinics have been set up in many hospitals. These clinics are staffed by various different specialists; surgeons, neurosurgeons and anaesthetists, and their aim is to offer special treatment for particular pain problems, not necessarily restricted to cancer-sufferers.

Nerves carrying pain from a particular area can be prevented from carrying these sensations by what is known as a nerve block. This is a procedure whereby either short- or long-acting local anaesthetics are injected into the nerves rendering them unable to carry pain sensation. Drugs such as alcohol or phenol can be used to permanently block nerves. As well as these local nerve blocks there are two methods of wholesale nerve blockage from an area such as the abdomen which is served by many nerves and the pain from which is necessarily diffuse.

The first of these is known as epidural anaesthesia. In this method a local anaesthetic is injected into the fluid surrounding the spinal cord so preventing the pain from reaching the central nervous system. Alternatively, a neurosurgeon can operate on the spinal cord and cut the nerve tracts within the spinal cord that are taking the sensation of pain to the brain.

As well as oral drugs to relieve pain and the various forms of neural block, both radiotherapy and chemotherapy can also be used to relieve pain. Radiotherapy is particularly useful for pain arising from bones, and radiotherapy and chemotherapy can treat pain by directly reducing the size of the cancerous mass that may be causing pain through direct expansion and pressure.

What is transcutaneous electrical nerve stimulation?

This form of pain relief is becoming increasingly widely available and can give real results. It entails placing two electrodes at specific sites over areas of cancer pain. The siting of these electrodes is crucially important but is normally a question of trial and error. A small direct current is then passed between the two electrodes giving a tingling sensation. This therapy does seem to offer a safe and effective method of treating some forms of cancer pain.

Can acupuncture therapy ease cancer pain?

Acupunture is a form of therapy that in the past has been considered to be outside orthodox medical treatment. It is politely termed an 'alternative' therapy because it is considered different to the traditional approach to the treatment of cancer pain.

Of late, however, it has been drawing more than just a passing interest from both patients and physicians because there are accumulating reports that, in certain circumstances, it has a role to play in the treatment of cancer pain.

There are a number of different forms of acupunture therapy but each specific one has as its basis the belief that there are specific small areas on or just beneath the skin that are neurologically connected with anatomical structures within the body. These specific points are connected by lines or meridians which can be traced on the body's skin, there being twelve main meridians.

The theory is that when specific anatomical structures become diseased, their acupuncture points become accentuated. This accentuation is recognized and then mapped out by the acupuncturist, and by mapping out points which, for instance, appear to be tender a diagnosis may be made.

Therapy is given by stimulating these acupuncture points either by simple pressure or by inserting fine needles into the skin at the sites of these points, stimulation being given by the needle or by electrical stimulation.

Currently, some scientists believe that by stimulating acupuncture points, natural chemicals within the brain called endorphins are released. It is thought that endorphins are naturally occurring pain-relieving chemicals and so cause the relief of pain in cancer in the best physiological way.

What problems can arise in the terminal phases of cancer?

Cancer is not the only illness with a terminal phase but one factor which distinguishes the terminal phase of cancer from that of some other diseases is the time span, which in some cases can be relatively protracted. Treatment of the cancer patient during this phase of his illness is just as important as the curative and palliative treatment that he will have already received.

Over the past decade there has been an increasing awareness within the medical profession of the importance of the treatment of cancer patients in the final, terminal phase of their illness. This phase is now much more actively spoken about and discussed.

As well as specific medication, an appreciation of the psychological changes in the patient is important because in such situations a patient's attitudes can often appear to be out of character and in some cases bizarre.

The patient's psychological reaction to terminal illness has been likened to the grief reaction that bereaved relatives often experience following the death of a family member. The patient may not consider the future, which can often incite a form of resentment in the patient's relatives. When they come to work through their grief reaction there is often the feeling that, in dying, the patient was thinking exclusively of himself at that time and not of the pain and suffering that those left behind would have to experience following his death.

This preoccupation with the present by the terminally ill patient can express itself in a number of different ways. For instance, if the patient is in hospital there may be an intense desire on his part to go home, just for an hour or two. There may be no particular point in going home but this is a desire that underlines a need to do something at that moment in time.

Psychologically a certain amount of depersonalization can result, wherever the terminal patient is being cared for, and this can often lead to symptoms of withdrawal. In some cases the feelings of depersonalization can be unwittingly created by the medical staff. For instance, in a hospital ward, conversations between medical staff can appear to the patient, not entirely relevant to his situation, lacking in any active help. Other patients may seem to be receiving more attention than the patient himself, so encouraging the patient to withdraw into himself. Compounding these feelings of isolation there is often a hidden guilt on the part of the patient about dying and leaving his relative behind. This can leave him feeling that he has let them down both financially and socially.

Such reactions and feelings can inevitably alter a patient's personality, something which is especially apparant to relatives. This change in personality can sometimes be most distressing for them because the ambivalence and latent anger that they perceive emanating from the dying patient excites a guilt reaction within them. They wonder if it is something they have said or done that has made their terminally ill relative appear distant and, in some cases, angry with them.

These are just a few examples of the psychological stresses and problems that beset both patients and relatives. It is essential that both medical staff and relatives appreciate that these problems exist. Without an understanding of these psychological situations, terminal care can often become even more distressing than it inevitably is.

Where should the terminally ill patient be cared for?

Probably the most important decision to be taken about terminal care is where the patient is to be nursed. There are three main possibilities, though a combination is often used.

The three areas in which care can be given are the home, a hospital or a hospice, and it should be stressed that care of the terminally ill patient should be no different in principle in any of these three locations. If there is no one to care for the patient at home or if the caring relative is too elderly or infirm to cope when members of the visiting medical team are not available, then hospitalization or hospice care is probably advisable. On the other hand, if the patient at home has able and willing relatives who can work with the visiting health care team, then both patient and relatives may decide that home care is the best alternative. The majority of patients in this country still die in hospital, the minority dying at home and in hospices. It is worth emphasizing, however, that the majority of these deaths in hospital include deaths not just from cancer but deaths from heart disease, lung disease, strokes and other illnesses. There is an increasing trend for patients with terminal cancer to be nursed either in hospices or at home or to spend part of the time in a hospice and part at home.

What is a hospice?

Hospices are centres for the care of the terminally ill; not necessarily cancer patients but also for patients with chronic illnesses such as multiple sclerosis and motor neurone disease.

Hospices have existed for many centuries, but it has only been since the 1950s that there has been a marked impetus in the hospice movement both in this country and abroad. In the vanguard of the hospice movement in the UK has been Dame Cicily Saunders who has blazed a trail with the organization and example of her hospice in the East End of London, St Joseph's Hospice.

The particular skill of those who work in hospices is in the assessment of the needs of the terminally ill patient and the best way in which to help the patient through their terminal illness.

Originally, hospice care was conducted on an in-patient basis but now such care is sometimes conducted on an outpatient basis, in which a team working from the hospice can care for a patient in his own home for a variable amount of time. The Macmillan nurses are a specially trained group of nurses who carry out this type of work.

In a hospice the medical team consists of doctors, nurses, physio-therapists, priests, social workers, and psychologists as well as voluntary workers. They work together with one purpose in mind: to bring physical and emotional comfort both to the terminally ill patient and his relatives.

One of the features which has left a lasting impression whenever I have visited a hospice is the cheerful atmosphere within it. You have to visit a hospice to appreciate this. They really are not the morbid places that you might imagine or expect. In the hospice, time is devoted to meeting all aspects of the patient's needs together with the family's needs – needs which, on the surface, may not appear important to the lay person but which are very important when caring for the terminally ill; for instance, the patient's appearance, his clothes and grooming. Then there is the general openness in the hospice, the patients being very much at the centre of activity rather than on the side-lines, as can happen in a general hospital ward. All these features may, to the lay person, seem unnecessary details but, to both the terminally ill patient and his relatives, they will inspire confidence; confidence both within themselves and within the hospice.

Pain is completely and continually treated though not to the extent of diminishing the patient's consciousness – a fine balance always being sought between the eradication of pain and maintaining alertness.

Terminal patients can experience a sensation of withdrawal and loneliness. The medical and nursing staff in the hospice will help to prevent these feelings and encourage the patient to look outwards.

What form of care can be given at home for the terminally ill patient?

This is an area with an overlap between a variety of services. In the past it was very much the province of the GP and today, in many areas, it still is. It is true that a caring GP who is known to both patient and family is probably the best person to cope with the terminally ill patient. Not only will he have known the family for some time but he will have been with the patient through the traumas of initial diagnosis and treatment and it is important for everybody that he be involved with the terminal care.

However, there is a growing problem in this respect. General practice, in some areas, is becoming less personalized. As practices grow larger it is often difficult to retain close continuity between a particular GP and a particular family.

Sometimes the needs of a terminally ill patient have to be met at night and that patient's particular doctor may not be on call on the night that he is most needed. In urban areas, where there is an increasing reliance upon deputizing services, a doctor unknown to the patient and his family may have to be called at this critical period. This can necessarily produce difficulties for both doctor and patient, and it is precisely because of these difficulties that the hospice system – consisting of staff based in a hospice but working mainly in the community (the Macmillan team) – has extended into the community.

With such services, a patient may be initially cared for at home. If terminal care problems become insurmountable then the patient can be transferred to the hospice while the home situation is sorted out. The patient may then return home and once more be looked after by the Macmillan team in the community. The care that the Macmillan service gives in the home is, of course, of the same nature and standard as that of the hospice care. It utilizes the same principles and practices of the hospice and so gives the patient the opportunity to be nursed at home during his illness.

What are the physical needs of a terminally ill patient?

Wherever the terminally ill patient is nursed, whether at home, in a hospice or in a hospital, there are a number of essential prerequisites to ensure adequate symptomatic treatment of his needs. Foremost amongst these needs is the adequate treatment of pain.

Constipation may also be a problem. This may be due to a number of factors, including the effects of the drugs used in pain therapy, and may in turn be exacerbated by lack of appetite and a reduced dietary intake. Treatment ranges from the use of mild laxatives which soften the stool and increase the bulk of the ingested material to more powerful ones which can be taken orally or as suppositories.

It is often the loss of appetite and the subsequent decrease in food intake in itself that is responsible for the constipation. This can be approached in a number of ways. One possibility is use of the steroid prednisolone, which stimulates the patient's appetite. Once this has been achieved, dietary intake will increase.

There may be other factors contributing to the poor dietary intake, however. It may, for example, be due to a sore mouth. The cancer itself and treatment such as chemotherapy can often reduce a patient's resistance to infection. It is often in the mouth that infection manifests itself in the form of ulcers in which fungal and viral infections flourish. Measures to reduce this problem are as follows. Basic dental hygiene is essential. This involves adequate cleaning of the teeth together with the use of mouth washes. In the case of fungal infections there are also a number of anti-fungal agents that can be taken either in tablet form or in the form of mouthwash. Sometimes the inability to take in food is due to serious problems such as vomiting. This can be controlled by the use of suitable medication, though sometimes the dehydration may become so severe that intravenous feeding is required.

Another problem that can be most troublesome is bladder control. The patient may suffer from urinary incontinence – an inability to retain urine. Alternatively, especially in men, urinary retention can cause considerable lower abdominal discomfort. In both circumstances urinary catherization may be useful. Equally, symptoms such as excessive coughing, breathlessness and symptoms of anaemia can all be medically corrected.

Although this list of problems may seem rather daunting, they can all be treated and no patient should have to suffer them.

Glossaries &
Useful Addresses

Glossary of Terms

Adenocarcinoma A cancerous change within glandular tissue.

Adenoma A benign tumour arising within glandular tissue.

Aflatoxin A carcinogenic substance produced by moulds.

Alopecia Hair loss.

Amenorrhoea Diminution or cessation of normal menstruation.

Anaemia A relative deficiency, or malfunctioning, of the red blood cells.

Analgesic Pain-relieving remedy.

Anaplastic A term used to describe immature or undifferentiated cells; it denotes rapidly growing cancer.

Anorexia The loss of appetite resulting in weight loss.

Antibody A protein that is part of the body's immune system. It neutralizes antigens.

Antigen A protein that is recognized by the body's immune system as being foreign to the body. Antigens encourage the production of antibodies.

Ascites The collection of fluid within the peritoneal cavity.

Aspiration The removal of excess fluid using a syringe.

Axilla The armpit.

Bacteria A single-celled micro-organism responsible for infection.

Basal cell carcinoma A skin cancer, also known as rodent ulcer.

Benign The term used to differentiate a state of non-cancerous tissue growth from cancerous tissue growth (malignant).

Biopsy The excision of tissue by surgical means for microscopic examination.

Bronchi The air passages connected to the lungs.

Bronchoscopy The examination of the bronchi by a bronchoscope.

Cachexia A state of generalized bodily wasting often seen in the terminal stages of cancer.

Carcinogen Any substance/chemical responsible for causing cancer.

Carcinoma A cancer arising from lining cells (otherwise known as epithelial cells).

Catheter A tube that can be introduced into any part of the body.

CAT scan Computerized tomography; a computer-directed X-ray examination.

Cerebrospinal fluid The fluid that bathes and surrounds the brain and the spinal cord.

Cervix The neck of the womb/uterus.

Chemotherapy   The treatment of cancer by the use of drugs.

Chromosome   A structure within the nucleus of the cell that is made up of units of proteins called genes.

Colostomy   An opening made through the abdominal wall through which the colon discharges faeces to the exterior.

Colposcopy   The examination of the cervix, via the vagina, using optical magnification.

Contrast medium   A radiological expression describing a substance that is opaque to X-rays.

Cyst   A benign swelling normally filled with fluid.

Cytology   The study of cells.

Cytotoxic   Any treatment that injures or kills cells (both normal and cancerous).

DNA   Deoxyribonucleic acid; a protein found within the chromosomes.

Dysplasia   The term used to describe abnormal-looking cells, though not necessarily with cancerous change.

Dysuria   Pain on urination.

Endocrine gland   A gland that produces and secretes hormones into the bloodstream.

Endometrium   The inner lining of the womb/uterus.

Endoscopy   The internal examination of an organ by use of an instrument (normally a fibre-optiscope).

Enzyme   A protein that speeds up chemical reactions.

Epidemiology   The study of disease within populations.

Epithelium   A thin layer of lining cells.

Gastroscopy   The examination of the internal aspect of the stomach with the use of a fibre-optiscope.

Gene   A section of a chromosome that carries hereditary information.

Glioma   A tumour of the central nervous system.

Haematuria   Blood in the urine.

Hepatoma   Cancer of the liver.

Hormone   A protein circulating in the blood, secreted by an endocrine gland. Hormones induce tissue changes.

Hospice   A special hospital for the care of the terminally ill.

Hysterectomy   The surgical removal of the uterus/womb.

Ileostomy   An opening within the abdominal wall through which the ileum (a part of the small intestine) is exteriorized, thereby allowing collection of intestinal waste matter.

Immunity   The process whereby the body protects itself from either infection or cancerous growth by the use of antibodies and white cells.

Immunotherapy   A technique whereby the body's immune system is stimulated to fight cancerous change.

Intravenous Term used to describe the introduction of a substance into a vein.

Laparotomy An exploratory abdominal operation.

Leukaemia A cancerous change in the white blood cells.

Lumbar puncture The introduction of a needle into the cerebrospinal fluid surrounding the spinal cord and removal of some of this fluid for laboratory examination.

Lymphangiogram The introduction of a radio-opaque substance into the body's lymphatic system with subsequent identification by X-rays.

Lymphatic system A connected series of channels through which lymph flows and is collected. These structures include the lymph vessels themselves, the spleen, the lymph nodes and the thymus gland.

Lymph node Small, circumscribed area of lymphatic tissue that produces lymphocytes.

Lymphocyte A sub-group of white cells.

Lymphoma A cancerous change arising in lymph nodes.

Malignant A term normally synonymous with cancerous change.

Mammography A low-dose X-ray examination of the breasts.

Mastectomy The surgical removal of the breast.

Melanoma A form of skin cancer.

Menopause The cessation of normal menstrual periods.

Mesothelioma A cancerous change arising from the pleura (lining of the lungs).

Metastasis The distant spread of cancerous tissue from the primary growth.

Mutation A change in the chemical configuration within a gene.

Myelography The introduction of a radio-opaque material into the cerebrospinal fluid; a subsequent X-ray examination may reveal structural faults.

Neoplasm The term used to describe new tissue growth; not necessarily cancerous.

Oestrogen A hormone secreted by the ovary.

Oncogene A section of genetic material capable of inducing cancerous change within tissues.

Oncology The study and treatment of cancer.

Oophorectomy The surgical removal of an ovary.

Orchidectomy The surgical removal of a testicle.

Pituitary gland An endocrine gland at the base of the brain that controls many of the body's other endocrine glands.

Platelet A blood cell, in part responsible for the clotting mechanism.

Pleura The external lining of the lungs.

Polyp A non-cancerous, balloon-like growth.

Progesterone A hormone produced by both the ovary and the placenta.

Prognosis A future view of the probability of the outcome of a disease.

Prosthesis An artificial replacement for a part of the body that has been removed.

Radiation Electromagnetic waves which may either be natural, as in ultraviolet radiation, or artificially produced, as in X-rays.

Radio-opaque A descriptive term for a substance that is opaque to X-ray.

Radiotherapy Treatment of cancerous tissue by electromagnetic radiation.

Remission The reduction or cessation of cancerous tissue growth.

Sarcoma A cancer arising in connective tissues, muscle and bone.

Sigmoidoscopy An examination of the sigmoid colon by use of a fibre-optiscope.

Staging A description of cancerous tissue in terms of spread.

Systemic A general term used to describe the whole body.

Tomogram A specialized and detailed form of X-ray study.

Tumour A very non-specific term that simply describes a swelling.

Ultrasound High-frequency sound waves that can identify solid structures within the body cavities.

Undifferentiated A description of rapidly dividing cancer cells denoting advanced and marked malignant change.

Vaccine A substance introduced into the body to stimulate an ability to provide immunity.

Virus The smallest of all known micro-organisms responsible for many types of infection.

X-ray High-energy electro-magnetic radiation.

Drug Glossary

CYTOTOXIC ANTIBIOTICS

BLEOMYCIN
ADMINISTRATION Intravenous.
USES Lymphoma; solid tumours.
POSSIBLE SIDE-EFFECTS Skin reactions: respiratory difficulties.

ACTINOMYCIN D
ADMINISTRATION Intravenous.
USES Children's cancers.
POSSIBLE SIDE-EFFECTS Bone marrow suppression; hair loss; nausea/vomiting.

DOXORUBICIN
ADMINISTRATION Intravenous.
USES Acute leukaemia; lymphoma.
POSSIBLE SIDE-EFFECTS Bone marrow suppression; hair loss; nausea/vomiting.

MITOMYCIN
ADMINISTRATION Intravenous.
USES Gastric, breast, oesophageal cancers.
POSSIBLE SIDE-EFFECTS Bone marrow suppression, lung and kidney damage.

ALKYLATING AGENTS

CHLORAMBUCIL
ADMINISTRATION Oral.
USES Chronic leukaemia; lymphoma; Hodgkin's disease; ovarian cancer.
POSSIBLE SIDE-EFFECTS Bone marrow suppression.

MELPHALAN
ADMINISTRATION Oral.
USES Multiple myeloma; lymphoma.
POSSIBLE SIDE-EFFECTS Bone marrow suppression.

CYCLOPHOSPHAMIDE
ADMINISTRATION Oral; intravenous.
USES Chronic lymphocytic leukaemia; lymphomas; solid tumours.
POSSIBLE SIDE-EFFECTS Urinary tract bleeding.

BUSULPHAN
ADMINISTRATION Oral.
USES Chronic myeloid leukaemia.
POSSIBLE SIDE-EFFECTS Bone marrow suppression; skin reactions.

LOMUSTINE
ADMINISTRATION Oral.
USES Hodgkin's disease.
POSSIBLE SIDE-EFFECTS Bone marrow suppression; nausea/vomiting.

THIOTEPA
ADMINISTRATION Directly into bladder/abdomen.
USES Bladder cancer; abdominal cancer.
POSSIBLE SIDE-EFFECTS Certain drug interactions.

ANTIMETABOLITES

CYTARABINE
ADMINISTRATION Intravenous.
USES Acute leukaemia.
POSSIBLE SIDE-EFFECTS Bone marrow suppression.

FLUOROURACIL
ADMINISTRATION Oral; intravenous.
USES Secondary spread from colonic cancer; breast cancer; skin cancer.
POSSIBLE SIDE-EFFECTS Bone marrow suppression.

METHOTREXATE
ADMINISTRATION Oral; intravenous; intramuscular.
USES Leukaemia; lymphoma; solid tumours.
POSSIBLE SIDE-EFFECTS Bone marrow suppression; kidney damage.

MECAPTOPURINE
ADMINISTRATION Oral.
USES Acute leukaemia.
POSSIBLE SIDE-EFFECTS Bone marrow suppression.

OTHER DRUGS

CISPLATIN
ADMINISTRATION Intravenous.
USES Ovarian cancer.
POSSIBLE SIDE-EFFECTS Bone marow suppression; nausea/ vomiting; kidney damage.

VINCRISTINE
ADMINISTRATION Intravenous.
USES Acute leukaemia; lymphoma; solid tumours.
POSSIBLE SIDE-EFFECTS Neuropathy; myopathy; hair loss.

VINBLASTINE
ADMINISTRATION Intravenous.
USES Lymphomas; solid tumours.
POSSIBLE SIDE-EFFECTS Bone marrow suppression.

HYDROXYUREA
ADMINISTRATION Oral.
USES Chronic leukaemia.
POSSIBLE SIDE-EFFECTS Bone marrow suppression; skin reactions.

PROCARBAZINE
ADMINISTRATION Oral.
USES Hodgkin's disease; lymphomas; lung cancer.
POSSIBLE SIDE-EFFECTS Bone marrow suppression; skin reactions.

HORMONE THERAPIES/HORMONE ANTAGONISTS

AMINOGLUTETHMIDE
ADMINISTRATION Oral.
USES Breast cancer.
POSSIBLE SIDE-EFFECTS Skin reactions.

STILBOESTROL
ADMINSTRATION Oral.
USES Post-menopausal breast cancer; prostate cancer.
POSSIBLE SIDE-EFFECTS Nausea; venous/arterial thromboses; impotence.

NORETHISTERONE
ADMINISTRATION Oral.
USES Breast cancer.
POSSIBLE SIDE-EFFECTS Nausea; fluid retention.

TAMOXIFEN
ADMINISTRATION Oral.
USES Breast cancer.
POSSIBLE SIDE-EFFECTS Few if any.

Useful addresses

British Association of Cancer United Patients
121/123 Charterhouse Street
London EC1M 6AA

Cancer Link
46 Pentonville Road
London N1 9HF

Cancer Research Campaign
2 Carlton House Terrace
London SW1Y 5AR

Imperial Cancer Research Fund
44 Lincoln's Inn Fields
London WC2A 3PX

Leukaemia Research Fund
43 Great Ormond Street
London WC1N 3JJ

Women's National Cancer Control Campaign
1 South Audley Street
London W1Y 5DQ

National Society for Cancer Relief
Anchor House
1519 Britten Street
London SW3 3TZ

Stoma Advisory Service
Abbot Laboratories Ltd.
Queensborough
Kent, ME11 5EL

Breast Care and Mastectomy Association
26 Harrison Street
London WC1H 8JG

Colostomy Welfare Group
38/39 Eccleston Square
London SW1V 1PB

Index

Index

INDEX